Diabetic Eye Disease

A Comprehensive Review

Diabetic Eye Disease

A Comprehensive Review

ALEJANDRO ESPAILLAT, MD
Director
Espaillat Vision & Clinical Research Network
Espaillat Diabetes Eye Care Foundation
Miami, Florida
Espaillat Eye & Laser Institute
Brickell Key Island, Miami, Florida
Laser Center at University of Miami Hospital
Miami, Florida

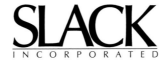

SLACK
INCORPORATED

ISBN: 978-1-61711-010-8

Published by: SLACK Incorporated
               6900 Grove Road
               Thorofare, NJ 08086 USA
               Telephone: 856-848-1000
               Fax: 856-848-6091
               www.slackbooks.com

Contact SLACK Incorporated for more information about other books in this field or about the availability of our books from distributors outside the United States.

Library of Congress Cataloging-in-Publication Data

Espaillat, Alejandro.
   Diabetic eye disease : a comprehensive review / Alejandro Espaillat.
     p. ; cm.
   Includes bibliographical references and index.
   ISBN 978-1-61711-010-8 (alk. paper)
   I. Title.
   [DNLM: 1. Diabetes Complications. 2. Eye Diseases--complications. 3. Diabetes Mellitus. WK 835]

617.7--dc23

2011043172

Printed in the United States of America

Last digit is print number: 10 9 8 7 6 5 4 3 2 1

DEDICATION

This book was conceived as a result of the personal interaction I had during my second year as a resident in ophthalmology, more than 15 years ago, with a diabetic patient under my care. During the postoperative period of an uneventful flawless cataract extraction, the patient complained of a painless sudden loss of vision on the operated eye. A detailed ophthalmic examination showed a central retinal vein occlusion as the etiology of the symptoms, and subsequent hand motion vision outcome. After such a dramatic experience, I promised myself to learn everything I could on how to better diagnose, treat, and prevent blindness from diabetic eye disease.

Many must be acknowledged, but I would like to particularly dedicate this book to the following:

- To the Massachusetts Eye & Ear Infirmary at Harvard Medical School, for teaching me that a clear and concise understanding of ophthalmic basic sciences is of paramount importance to becoming a great eye clinician and surgeon.
- To the Carney Hospital, Internal Medicine Department, Boston University School of Medicine, for teaching me how systemic diseases could also have a significant impact on the organ of vision.
- To the entire ophthalmology department, at the Rhode Island Hospital, Brown University School of Medicine, for training me to become an eye physician and surgeon.
- To the Joslin Diabetes Center, Beetham Eye Institute, Harvard Medical School; particularly Dr. Lloyd M. Aiello and Dr. Lloyd P. Aiello, for teaching that the only way to treat a systemic disease is applying a multidisciplinary approach mostly at one location.
- To the American Diabetes Association, for supporting and funding my clinical research on cataract surgery on diabetic patients.
- To the National Diabetes Institute, Santo Domingo, Dominican Republic, for granting me the possibility to teach for 1 year, and care for poorly controlled diabetic patients. I will never forget the amazing experience it was caring for these poorly treated and underserved patients, while giving back some of the advanced training acquired to the country I was born.
- To the University of Miami Hospital medical staff and administration, in particular to Mr. Luis del Pozo, for supporting my efforts when caring for our community of patients.
- To Dr. Camillo Ricordi, scientific director at the Diabetes Research Institute, Miami, Florida. His amazing work generates shock waves among the diabetes scientific community; defeating the disease, and granting years of life to diabetic patients around the globe.
- To Dr. Pascal Goldschmidt, dean of the University of Miami School of Medicine, for his wide angle academic vision, leadership, and extraordinary work on the diagnosis and new treatment modalities on the cardiovascular manifestations of diabetes mellitus.
- To my mother and sisters, as well as to my father, for his over 40 years as an Ophthalmologist caring for the diabetic patient in the Dominican Republic.
- To my brother, for his outstanding work as an educator, medical director, and eye physician surgeon caring for diabetic patients in Santo Domingo, Dominican Republic.
- And finally, to Rosanna, and my children, Veronica and Marco, for their invaluable support and unconditional love during my life's journey.

CONTENTS

About the Author

Alejandro Espaillat, MD is an eye physician specialized on state-of-the-art anterior segment surgery and diabetic eye disease. He is an active eye surgeon who has performed thousands of small incision refractive cataract extractions and laser ophthalmic surgeries. He has spent most of his years in practice caring for patients affected by diabetic eye disease.

Dr. Espaillat has participated in the research and co-authorship of many published scientific medical reports, has designed surgical instruments used during cataract surgeries, and has lectured extensively nationally and internationally on the topic of diabetic eye disease, particularly the management of cataract surgery on the diabetic patient.

Dr. Espaillat is in private practice in Miami, Florida, as the medical director of the Espaillat Eye & Laser Institute, Espaillat Vision & Clinical and Research Network, and chairman of his own nonprofit Diabetes Eye Care Foundation.

Contributing Authors

Lloyd M. Aiello, MD *(Chapter 9)*
Founding Director, Beetham Eye Institute
Joslin Diabetes Center
Clinical Professor, Department of Ophthalmology
Harvard Medical School
Boston, Massachusetts

Lloyd Paul Aiello, MD, PhD *(Chapter 9)*
Director, Beetham Eye Institute
Head, Section Eye Research
Joslin Diabetes Center
Associate Professor, Department of Ophthalmology
Harvard Medical School
Boston, Massachusetts

Larissa Camejo, MD *(Chapter 6)*
Assistant Professor of Ophthalmology
University of Pittsburgh
Pittsburgh, Pennsylvania

Jerry D. Cavallerano, OD, PhD *(Chapter 9)*
Beetham Eye Institute
Joslin Diabetes Center
Associate Professor, Department of Ophthalmology
Harvard Medical School
Boston, Massachusetts

Sandra Rocio Montezuma, MD *(Chapter 8)*
Assistant Professor of Ophthalmology
Department of Ophthalmology
University of Minnesota
Minneapolis, Minnesota

Timothy J. Murtha, MD *(Chapter 5)*
Eye Physician and Surgeon
Beetham Eye Institute
Joslin Diabetes Center
Harvard Medical School
Boston, Massachusetts

Deval (Reshma) Paranjpe, MD *(Chapter 3)*
Assistant Professor of Ophthalmology
Drexel University College of Medicine
Director, Cornea and External Disease Service
Department of Ophthalmology
Allegheny General Hospital
Pittsburgh, Pennsylvania

Roberto Pineda, MD *(Chapter 4)*
Director of Refractive Surgery
Massachusetts Eye and Ear Infirmary
Assistant Professor of Ophthalmology
Harvard Medical School
Boston, Massachusetts

Jesse Richman, MD *(Chapter 6)*
Chief Resident
Department of Ophthalmology
Rhode Island Hospital
Brown University School of Medicine
Providence, Rhode Island

Susannah G. Rowe, MD, MPH *(Chapter 2)*
Assistant Professor of Ophthalmology
Director, Patient Safety and Quality
Vice Chair for Finance
Department of Ophthalmology
Boston University School of Medicine
Boston Medical Center
Boston, Massachusetts

Cecilia R. Sanchez, MD *(Chapter 5)*
Ophthalmology Clinical Fellow
Beetham Eye Institute
Joslin Diabetes Center
Harvard Medical School
Boston, Massachusetts

Evana Valenzuela Scheker, MD *(Chapter 1)*
Diabetes Eye Care Institute
University of Miami Hospital
Miami, Florida

Sabera T. Shah, MD *(Chapter 5)*
Eye Physician and Surgeon
Beetham Eye Institute
Joslin Diabetes Center
Harvard Medical School
Boston, Massachusetts

Paolo S. Silva, MD *(Chapter 9)*
Assistant Chief, Center for Ocular Telehealth
Beetham Eye Institute
Joslin Diabetes Center
Instructor in Ophthalmology
Harvard Medical School
Boston, Massachusetts

King To, MD *(Chapter 6)*
Department of Ophthalmology
Rhode Island Hospital
Clinical Professor of Ophthalmology
Brown University School of Medicine
Providence, Rhode Island

Dorothy Tolls, OD *(Chapter 9)*
Beetham Eye Institute
Joslin Diabetes Center
Boston, Massachusetts

Glenn C. Yiu, MD, PhD (Chapter 8)
Ophthalmology Resident
Massachusetts Eye & Ear Infirmary
Clinical Fellow in Ophthalmology
Harvard Medical School
Boston, Massachusetts

PREFACE

Writing a comprehensive, practical, easy to read, and up-to-date book on the potential ophthalmic manifestations caused by diabetes mellitus has been a project I have had in mind for over 10 years. Detailed descriptions on the epidemiology, diagnosis, laboratory tests, and treatment alternatives are made available to all health care providers, but particularly to those caring for the diabetic patient.

Thanks to the efforts of the superb chapter authors, and the extraordinary publishing staff at SLACK Incorporated, this book is now a reality available to all.

Respectfully penned,
Alejandro Espaillat, MD
Miami, Florida

1

Diabetes Mellitus
Diagnosis and Current and Future Therapies

Evana Valenzuela Scheker, MD and Alejandro Espaillat, MD

Diabetes mellitus is defined as a syndrome characterized by hyperglycemia resulting from absolute or relative impairment in insulin secretion and/or insulin action.

It is the most common endocrine disease, causing metabolic abnormalities and long-term complications involving the eyes, kidneys, nerves, and blood vessels.[1]

The most prominent effects of insulin are the stimulation of glucose uptake by peripheral tissues (mainly skeletal muscle) and the suppression of endogenous glucose production (predominately hepatic glycogenolysis and gluconeogenesis). In addition, insulin suppresses lipolysis in adipocytes and proteolysis in muscle. In healthy people, glucose concentrations are kept within a relatively narrow range by low concentrations of insulin during fasting (to suppress hepatic glucose production) and exuberant spikes of insulin during meals (to dispose of glucose into cells).[2]

CLASSIFICATION

In 1997, the American Diabetes Association (ADA) issued a new diagnostic and classification criteria; in 2003, modifications were made regarding the diagnosis of impaired fasting glucose. The classification of diabetes includes 4 clinical classes:

1. *Type 1 diabetes*: Mainly affects children, teenagers, and young adults. It is characterized by an absolute insulin deficiency from selective autoimmune destruction of the pancreatic beta cells. The disorder has a strong genetic association with major histocompatibility complex human leukocyte antigen (HLA) DQA and DQB.[3]

2. *Type 2 diabetes*: Results from a progressive insulin secretory defect on the background of insulin resistance. The typical patient is older than age 40 and overweight, accounting for more than 90% of patients suffering from diabetes. Due to the rise in obesity, type 2 diabetes is seen more frequently in a younger population (children and teenagers). Patients with insulin resistance do not develop diabetes if their β-cell function is preserved.

   The co-occurrence of metabolic risk factors for both type 2 diabetes and cardiovascular disease (CVD; abdominal obesity, hyperglycemia, dyslipidemia, and hypertension) suggested the existence of a "metabolic syndrome."

3. *Gestational diabetes mellitus*: Diabetes diagnosed during pregnancy.

4. *Other*: Genetic defects in β-cell function, genetic defects in insulin action, diseases of the exocrine pancreas (such as cystic fibrosis), and drug or chemical induced.

Espaillat A.
Diabetic Eye Disease: A Comprehensive Review (pp. 1-10)
© 2012 SLACK Incorporated

Table 1-1. Diagnosis Criteria for Diabetes and Pre-diabetes States

Diagnosis	Fasting Plasma Glucose	Casual Plasma Glucose	2-hour Oral Plasma Glucose
Normal glucose homeostasis	<100 mg/dL		<140 mg/dL
Impaired glucose homeostasis ("pre-diabetes")	100 to 125 mg/dL (impaired fasting glucose)		140 to 199 mg/dL (impaired glucose tolerance)
Diabetes*	≥126 mg/dL	≥200mg/dL Plus symptoms of hyperglycemia	≥200 mg/dL

*In the absence of unequivocal hyperglycemia, these criteria should be confirmed by repeat testing on a different day.

Adapted from the American Diabetes Association. Standards of medical care in diabetes—2009. *Diabetes Care.* 2009;32(suppl 1):S13-S61.

Some patients cannot be clearly classified as having type 1 or type 2 diabetes. Clinical presentation and disease progression may vary in both types of diabetes. Occasionally, patients who otherwise have type 2 diabetes may present with ketoacidosis; similarly, patients with type 1 diabetes may have a late onset and slow, but relentless, progression of the disease despite having features of autoimmune disease. Such difficulties in diagnosis may occur in children, adolescents, and adults. The true diagnosis may become more obvious over time.[1]

DIAGNOSIS

Signs and symptoms of osmotic diuresis and hyperglycemia make the diagnosis unequivocal, as well as an asymptomatic patient with elevated fasting plasma glucose concentrations.

The classical signs of hyperglycemia include polyuria, polydipsia, and unexplained weight loss.

The ADA and World Health Organization have established the following criteria for the diagnosis of diabetes:

- Impaired fasting glucose, in which the fasting plasma glucose (FPG) level is between 100 and 125 mg/dL
- Oral glucose tolerance test (OGTT), in which the glucose level reaches 140 to 199 mg/dL 2 hours after a 75-g oral glucose load.[1,2,4]

Patients with impaired fasting glucose or impaired OGTT are at higher risk for the future development of diabetes.[1,5]

Although the OGTT is not recommended for routine clinical use, it may be useful for further evaluation of patients in whom diabetes is still strongly suspected but who have normal FPG or impaired fasting glucose.[1]

If a patient meets the diabetes criteria of the glycohemoglobin (HbA1C—2 results ≥6.5%) but not the FPG (<126 mg/dL), or vice versa, he or she should be considered to have diabetes. Admittedly, in most circumstances, the "nondiabetic" test is likely to be in a range very close to the threshold that defines diabetes (Table 1-1).[6,7]

Historically, the HbA1C test has been recommended only for the determination of glucose control among persons who have already received the diagnosis of diabetes, in part due to lack of standardization of the assay. However, A1C assays are now highly standardized so that their results can be uniformly applied both temporally and across populations. New ADA clinical practice recommendations advocate the use of HbA1C in the diagnosis of diabetes, largely on the basis of the established association between HbA1C and microvascular disease. The current recommendation in the use of the HbA1C test to diagnose diabetes is a threshold of ≥6.5%. The diagnostic HbA1C cutoff point of 6.5% is associated with an inflection point for retinopathy prevalence, as are the diagnostic thresholds for FPG and 2-hour OGTT. Compared with fasting glucose, HbA1C has several advantages as a diagnostic test: it has higher repeatability, can be assessed in the nonfasting state,[8-11] and is the preferred test for monitoring glucose control.

The diagnostic test should be performed using a method that is certified by the National Glycohemoglobin Standardization Program and standardized or traceable to the Diabetes Control and Complications Trial reference assay.[11]

COMPLICATIONS

Acute Complications

Diabetic Ketoacidosis

The most life-threatening acute complication of diabetes, and often the presenting manifestation of type 1 diabetes, is diabetic ketoacidosis (DKA). The major manifestations are hyperglycemia, ketosis, and dehydration, which are directly or indirectly related to insulin deficiency. The lack of insulin prevents glucose uptake by muscle and allows unrestrained hepatic glucose production. Lack of suppression of lipolysis also leads to excess free fatty acids, which are converted to ketoacids by the liver.

- *Clinical presentation*: History of polyuria, polydipsia, and blurred vision, followed by nausea, vomiting, abdominal pain, dyspnea, and altered mental status.
- *Management*: Aggressive hydration, intravenous insulin, and electrolyte repletion.

Hyperglycemic Hyperosmolar Syndrome

This syndrome occurs in patients with type 2 diabetes. As opposed to DKA, this condition lacks significant metabolic acidosis. The treatment is similar to DKA.[12]

Hypoglycemia

Hypoglycemia, defined as a plasma glucose concentration <60 mg/dL, in diabetes is typically the result of the interplay of absolute or relative therapeutic insulin excess and compromised physiological and behavioral defenses against falling plasma glucose concentrations. The protective response to hypoglycemia is impaired in most patients with type 1 diabetes and in many patients with long-standing type 2 diabetes. Hypoglycemia causes a vicious cycle of recurrent autonomic failure.

Hypoglycemia usually occurs after missed meals, excessive exercise, alcohol use, or excessive insulin administration. The initial signs are related to a hyperadrenergic state including diaphoresis, tachycardia, anxiety, and tremor. When the blood glucose drops between 40 and 50 mg/dL, neuroglycopenic signs and symptoms develop such as personality change, cognitive impairment, loss of consciousness, and seizures. In severe cases, coma and irreversible brain injury may occur.

Most episodes of severe hypoglycemia occur during sleep, with multiple factors playing a role. It is the longest interprandial period, and sympathoadrenal responses to hypoglycemia are also reduced during sleep.

Hypoglycemia is reversible after ingestion or administration of carbohydrates such as glucose- or sucrose-containing foods, intravenous dextrose infusion, or intramuscular glucagon.

It remains the most important impediment to achieving tight glycemic control in insulin-treated patients.[13]

Chronic Complications

1. *Microvascular disease*: Involves the kidneys (diabetic nephropathy), retinae (diabetic retinopathy), and peripheral nerves (diabetic neuropathy).
2. *Macrovascular disease*: Involves the coronary, carotid, and cerebral arteries; the aorta; and the arterial supply to the legs.

Patients with type 2 diabetes more commonly have macrovascular complications because of generally older age and the frequent coexistence of other cardiovascular risk factors such as obesity, hypertension, and lipid disorders.[14]

Diabetic Nephropathy

Diabetic nephropathy is one of the most common causes of renal failure. Abnormal albumin excretion is an early sign of glomerular disease and may progress slowly from microalbuminuria to macroalbuminuria. Albumin and creatinine are measured annually. The progression of the disease is halted by blood pressure control, mainly by modulating the renin-angiotensin-aldosterone axis with angiotensin-converting enzyme (ACE) inhibitors or angiotensin-II receptor blockers, and glucose control.[15]

Diabetic Neuropathy

Diabetes injures sensory, motor, and autonomic nerves. The most common presentation is the loss of sensation in the lower extremities, which contributes to foot ulceration. Patients may also present with erectile dysfunction, orthostatic hypotension, gastroparesis, diabetic diarrhea, and atonic bladder. Improving glucose control is the only direct treatment for the neuropathy, but it does not alleviate the symptoms of autonomic neuropathy.[16] Pharmacological therapy helps ameliorate the symptoms, including tricyclic antidepressants, capsaicin, gabapentin, and pregabalin, among others.

Foot Care

Diabetic patients need an annual comprehensive foot examination to identify the risk factors predictive of ulcers and amputations. The risk for the above are previous amputation, past foot ulcers, peripheral neuropathy,

Table 1-2. American Diabetes Association Lipid Guidelines

Assessment	Goal	Drug Therapy Initiation
LDL-C		
With CVD	<100 mg/dL	>100 mg/dL
	<70 mg/dL in very high-risk patients	
Without CVD	<100 mg/dL	>100 mg/dL
HDL-C	>40 mg/dL (men)	No guidelines
	>50 mg/dL (women)	
TG	<150 mg/dL	>400 mg/dL

foot deformity, peripheral vascular disease, vision impairment, diabetic nephropathy (especially dialysis), poor glycemic control, and cigarette smoking.

Cardiovascular Disease

The risk of CVD increases 2- to 4-fold in patients with diabetes. The presence of diabetes is a cardiovascular risk equivalent. The detrimental effects of hyperglycemia and hyperinsulinemia include hypertension, dyslipidemia, endothelial cell dysfunction, hypercoagulability, and vascular inflammation.

- *Hypercoagulability*: The prevention of CVD includes aspirin to decrease platelet hyperaggregability. The dose is 75 to 162 mg/d as primary and secondary prevention. It is not recommended in patients younger than 30 years of age due to lack of evidence of benefits and is contraindicated in patients younger than 21 years of age because of the associated risk of Reye's syndrome. Low-dose aspirin is a "reasonable" choice for adults with diabetes who have a 10-year risk for CVD >10% and are not at increased risk for bleeding.[17]

- *Blood pressure control*: Another critical part of the prevention of CVD is blood pressure control, which ideally should be below 130/80 mm Hg.[18] Hypertension treatment begins with lifestyle modifications for a maximum of 3 months if blood pressure is <140/90 mm Hg; if the targets are not achieved, pharmacological agents will be added, among them ACE inhibitors and angiotensin receptor blocker, which also slow the progression of renal disease.

- *Lipid management*: The ADA recommends screening for lipid disorders at least annually in patients with diabetes, and more often if needed to achieve goals. Adults with low-risk lipid values (low-density lipoprotein [LDL] <100 mg/dL, high-density lipoprotein [HDL] >50 mg/dL, and

triglycerides [TG] <150 mg/dL) may be screened every 2 years. Table 1-2 shows the ADA guidelines for lipid management.

Lipid management is achieved by lifestyle modifications focusing on the reduction of saturated fat, trans fat, and cholesterol intake; weight loss; increased physical activity; and smoking cessation. If goals are not met, then pharmacological therapy is initiated. The priority for lipid management is first to lower LDL level, then to raise HDL concentration, and finally to lower the TG levels. The preferred drugs for lipid management are statins (they have the highest impact on lowering LDL levels), followed by cholesterol absorption inhibitors, binding resins, fenofibrates (raise HDL and lower TG), or niacin (raise HDL).

If a patient is >40 years old, with at least one additional CVD risk factor, statin therapy is started to achieve an LDL reduction of 30% to 40% regardless of baseline LDL. If the patient is younger than 40 years, statin therapy should be considered to achieve LDL levels <100 mg/dL if he or she is at increased risk due to other CVD risk factors or long duration of diabetes.[19]

- *Smoking cessation*: Diabetic patients should be counseled for smoking cessation, as it increases the risk of CVD and premature death. It is also related to the premature development of microvascular complications of diabetes and may have a role in the development of type 2 diabetes.[20]

Infections

Patients with diabetes are considered immunosuppressed and exhibit an increased predisposition to infections.[21] Neutrophil chemotaxis and adherence to vascular endothelium, phagocytosis, intracellular bactericidal activity, opsonization, and cell-mediated immunity are all depressed in diabetics with hyperglycemia. The most common infections are candidiasis, mucormycosis, and necrotizing external otitis.

Glucose-inducible proteins promote adhesion of *Candida albicans* to buccal or vaginal epithelium.[22] This adhesion impairs phagocytosis, giving the organism an advantage over the host.

Ketone reductases allow *Rhizopus spp.*[23] to thrive in high glucose, acidic conditions typically present in diabetic patients with ketoacidosis.

TREATMENT

The ADA advises tight glucose control in patients with diabetes. The recommended HbA1C should be <6.5%, preprandial plasma glucose between 90 and 130 mg/dL, and postprandial plasma glucose of <180 mg/dL.[24]

The most reliable assessment of overall glycemic status is the periodic measurement of the HbA1C. It determines the average degree of glycemia over the previous 2 to 3 months. Frequent capillary glucose monitoring is helpful and a more immediate adjunct to the HbA1C measurement. Plasma glucose should be kept between 90 and 120 mg/dL before meals and <180 mg/dL 2 hours after meals.[25]

Patient education and self-management training are critical in diabetes therapy, regarding glucose monitoring techniques, insulin and oral agent administration, treatment of hypoglycemia, and when to seek medical care.

Type 1 Diabetes Mellitus

The Diabetes Control and Complications Trial and other smaller studies demonstrated that improved glycemic control with intensive insulin therapy in patients with type 1 diabetes mellitus led to significant reductions in retinopathy, nephropathy, and neuropathy. Intensive insulin therapy also reduces cardiovascular morbidity and mortality.[26]

Intensive therapy should be started as soon as the diagnosis of type 1 diabetes is made, which slows the loss of B-cell function, reduces the risk for retinopathy progression, and lowers the risk for severe hypoglycemia.

The choice of insulin depends on patient and physician preference. The basic requirements are a stable baseline dose of intermediate or long-acting insulin in addition to concomitant pre-meal use of short-acting insulin. Most patients with type 1 diabetes require between 0.5 and 1.0 units of insulin per kilogram of body weight per day.

Nocturnal hypoglycemia is common in patients with type 1 diabetes treated with twice daily insulin.[27]

Type 2 Diabetes Mellitus

Improving the glycemic control in type 2 diabetes lessens the risk of microvascular complications but does not alter the macrovascular outcomes. It is treated initially with diet (caloric restriction), weight loss, and exercise. Bariatric surgery for weight loss treatment of morbidly obese patients with diabetes results in the largest degree of sustained weight loss and the largest improvements in blood glucose control. Such lifestyle modifications reduce insulin resistance, blood glucose levels, and cardiovascular complications. Most patients are started on oral agents after lifestyle modifications alone fail to normalize the glucose level.[25]

Metformin therapy should be initiated, concurrent with lifestyle modifications, at the time of diagnosis according to the ADA and the European Association for the Study of Diabetes. In patients with contraindications to metformin, sulfonylureas are recommended.

In 2009, rosiglitazone was contraindicated due to findings related to increased cardiovascular risk and congestive heart failure.

A combination of different agents usually is necessary to achieve optimal results.

Metformin

As previously mentioned, metformin is the first choice for oral treatment. It lowers HbA1C by 1.5% points.[28] Unlike other agents, monotherapy with metformin does not usually cause hypoglycemia. It is effective only in the presence of insulin, and its major effect is to decrease hepatic glucose output. It increases insulin-mediated glucose utilization in peripheral tissues (such as muscle and liver), particularly after meals, and has an antilipolytic effect that lowers serum free fatty acid concentrations, thereby reducing substrate availability for gluconeogenesis. As a result of the improvement in glycemic control, serum insulin concentrations decline slightly.[29]

Metformin has lipid-lowering activity, resulting in a decrease in serum TG and free fatty acid concentrations, a small decrease in serum LDL cholesterol concentrations, and a very modest increase in serum HDL cholesterol concentrations.

Gastrointestinal side effects are common, including a metallic taste in the mouth, mild anorexia, nausea, abdominal discomfort, and soft bowel movements or diarrhea.[29,30]

It can rarely cause lactic acidosis and therefore should not be administered when conditions predisposing to lactic acidosis are present, including impaired renal function, decreased tissue perfusion, hemodynamic instability, liver disease, or heart failure. Patients undergoing a surgical procedure or intravenous iodinated contrast material should have metformin suspended until renal function and circulation can be evaluated.

Metformin was associated with fewer episodes of hypoglycemia compared with sulfonylureas and less edema, congestive heart failure, and weight gain compared with thiazolidinediones. It reduces intestinal absorption of vitamin B_{12} and lowers serum vitamin B_{12} concentration, but rarely causes megaloblastic anemia.[29,31]

Sulfonylureas

Glyburide, glipizide, and glimepiride are considered insulin secretagogues. They bind to the sulfonylurea receptor on the beta cell, closing adenosine triphosphate (ATP)-dependent potassium channels and leading to depolarization of the cell membrane. The net effect is increased responsiveness of β cells to both glucose and nonglucose secretagogues (eg, amino acids), resulting in more insulin being released at all blood glucose concentrations. Circulating insulin concentrations increase, partly overcoming peripheral insulin resistance. They lower blood glucose concentrations by 20% and HbA1C by 1% to 2%. However, effectiveness decreases over time.

The major side effect is hypoglycemia. Patients should be advised about the signs and symptoms of hypoglycemia prior to starting treatment with sulfonylureas. Risk factors for hypoglycemia include increasing age, alcohol abuse, poor nutrition, and renal insufficiency. Shorter-acting sulfonylureas are less likely to cause hypoglycemia. Sulfonylureas are also associated with weight gain. Other infrequent side effects include nausea, skin reaction, and abnormal liver function tests.

Some studies suggest that sulfonylureas may be associated with poorer outcomes after a myocardial infarction, including the University Group Diabetes Study against tolbutamide; a study at Mayo Clinic following diabetic patients undergoing percutaneous coronary intervention; and the Diabetes Mellitus Insulin Glucose Infusion in Acute Myocardial Infarction (DIGAMI), where the patients with the poorest outcome were those treated with sulfonylurea at the time of the myocardial infarction.[32]

It is possible that the presence of sulfonylureas during a myocardial infarction prevents adequate coronary vasodilation and thus may result in a larger area of damage. The newer sulfonylureas are more pancreatic selective. Newer clinical trials such as the Action in Diabetes and Vascular Disease (ADVANCE) are somewhat reassuring, although they are not specifically designed to address this issue.[33]

Meglitinides

Repaglinide and nateglinide are short-acting, glucose-lowering drugs that act similarly to sulfonylureas and have similar or slightly less efficacy in decreasing glycemia. They are structurally different than sulfonylurea and utilize different receptors but also regulate the ATP-dependent potassium channels in pancreatic β cells.[34]

Repaglinide reduces the HbA1C further than nateglinide. Repaglinide has similar efficacy in reducing HbA1C values as metformin.

Repaglinide could be considered as initial therapy in patients with chronic kidney disease who are intolerant of sulfonylureas. Hypoglycemia is the most common side effect.

Thiazolidinediones

Rosiglitazone and pioglitazone lower blood concentrations by increasing insulin sensitivity. They increase insulin sensitivity by acting on adipose, muscle, and liver to increase glucose utilization and decrease glucose production. They may also improve blood glucose levels by preserving pancreatic B-cell function.

As monotherapy, they lower HbA1C by 0.5% to 1.4%. They appear to be more effective when used in combination therapy with an agent that has a different mechanism of action.

They are contraindicated in patients with New York Heart Association class III or IV heart failure. Some analysts have questioned the safety of rosiglitazone with regard to the risk of myocardial infarction and atherogenic lipid profile. Meta-analyses demonstrated a small increase in myocardial infarction in patients using rosiglitazone. Previously, the Rosiglitazone Evaluated for Cardiovascular Outcomes and Regulation of Glycaemia in Diabetes (RECORD) found an increased risk of fatal and nonfatal heart failure in patients consuming this agent.[35]

Additionally, pioglitazone produces a more favorable lipid profile. Decreases in TG levels were observed more often with pioglitazone than with rosiglitazone, as well as a milder increase in LDL concentration. If thiazolidinediones are initiated, the recommended second-line agent should be pioglitazone.[36]

Thiazolidinediones are also associated with more weight gain and fluid retention than metformin. The fluid retention is more prominent with concomitant insulin therapy. This fluid retention may lead to or worsen heart failure. Macular edema has been reported, although the frequency of occurrence is unknown.

Glucagon-like Peptide 1 Agonists

The glucagon-like peptide-1 (GLP-1) exerts its main effect by stimulating glucose-dependent insulin release from the pancreatic islets. It also slows gastric emptying, inhibits inappropriate postmeal glucagon release, and reduces food intake.[37]

The United States Food and Drug Administration approved exenatide and liraglutide for the treatment of type 2 diabetes in patients not sufficiently controlled with diet, exercise, or oral agents.

Exenatide is a GLP-1 analogue resistant to dipeptidyl peptidase IV (DPP-IV) degradation. It exhibits dose-dependent and glucose-dependent augmentation of insulin secretion. It is approved for monotherapy or in combination with oral agents. It decreases HbA1C by 1%. It is associated with weight loss and subsequent improvement in blood pressure and lipids.[38] Exenatide is not currently approved for use with insulin therapy. The most common side effects are gastrointestinal, predominantly nausea. Other less common side effects are pancreatitis and acute renal failure.[39]

Liraglutide is a GLP-1 analogue modified for slower degradation. It also decreases HbA1C by 1%. As exenatide, it is also associated with significant weight loss. The most common side effects are nausea, vomiting, and diarrhea. In a trial comparing both GLP-1 analogues, a greater reduction of HbA1C was reported in patients taking liraglutide than exenatide.[40]

Dipeptidyl Peptidase IV Inhibitor

DPP-IV is a ubiquitous enzyme expressed on the surface of most cell types that deactivates a variety of bioactive peptides, including gastrointestinal peptides (GIP) and GLP-1, affecting glucose regulation.

Sitagliptin usually is used as a second- or third-line agent. It decreases HbA1C by 0.6%. It may be considered as monotherapy in patients intolerant to metformin, sulfonylureas, or thiazolidinediones, or in combination with the above-mentioned agents. There are no effects on body weight or hypoglycemia risk. Increased risk is present for pancreatitis and skin hypersensitivity reactions. Saxagliptin is another drug of this group that has a profile similar to sitagliptin.[41]

Alpha-Glucosidase Inhibitors

These inhibitors lower the blood glucose by modifying the intestinal absorption of carbohydrates, inhibiting the upper gastrointestinal enzymes (alpha-glucosidases) that convert carbohydrates into monosaccharides in a dose-dependent fashion. The slower rise in postprandial blood glucose concentration is potentially beneficial in both type 1 and type 2 diabetes. It may also increase insulin sensitivity in older patients with type 2 diabetes.

Acarbose and miglitol have additive hypoglycemic effects in patients on concomitant sulfonylurea, metformin, or insulin therapy. They lower the HbA1C by 0.5% to 0.8%.

The main side effects are flatulence and diarrhea. They do not cause weight gain. There are no studies comparing both drugs against each other.[42]

In one study, acarbose therapy reduced the risk of cardiovascular events by 49% when compared to placebo. The major reduction was in myocardial infarction. Decreasing postprandial hyperglycemia in patients with impaired glucose tolerance may lower the risk of CVD and hypertension.[43]

Lipase Inhibitors

Orlistat is a minimally absorbed drug that inhibits pancreatic and gastric lipases, blocking absorption of approximately 30% of ingested fat. The main effect is weight loss, which can improve glucose tolerance and slow the rate of progression to type 2 diabetes. A trial with orlistat showed that patients taking this drug had a greater decrease in serum total cholesterol and LDL cholesterol concentrations compared to placebo. Orlistat may be a useful adjunct therapy for patients with type 2 diabetes (Table 1-3).[44]

Insulin

In patients with type 2 diabetes, insulin usually is started when inadequate glycemic control persists despite treatment with oral agents and lifestyle modification. There are increasing data that more aggressive use of insulin may be beneficial. Insulin requirements are greater in patients with type 2 diabetes as compared to type 1. Insulin lowers the HbA1C by 1.5% to 2.5%.

Insulin is the preferred second-line medication for patients with HbA1C >8.5% or with symptoms of hyperglycemia despite metformin titration.

Insulin is secreted in a pulsatile fashion with a basal level under unstimulated conditions and also in response to meals. Basal insulin represents 50% of the insulin production.[45]

Intensive insulin therapy describes the regimens in which a more physiologic approach is taken, with a basal insulin delivery and superimposed doses of short-acting insulin. These regimens were first established for type 1 diabetics, but are now used for type 2 diabetics as well.

Intensive insulin therapy is generally provided in 2 ways:

1. As a basal supplement with an intermediate to long-acting preparation to suppress hepatic glucose production and maintain a near normoglycemic fasting state.

2. As a prandial bolus dose of short- or rapid-acting insulin to cover the extra requirements after food is absorbed (Table 1-4 and Figure 1-1).[45-47]

Table 1-3. Oral Agents for Type 2 Diabetes

Medications	Hemoglobin A1C Change (%)	Mechanism of Action	Benefits	Risks/Side Effects
Metformin	1 to 2	Decreases hepatic glucose production	Weight loss; lipid profile improvement; improves macrovascular outcomes; no hypoglycemia	Lactic acidosis; diarrhea; lowers B_{12} levels
Sulfonylureas	1 to 2	Binds to sulfonylurea receptor, stimulating insulin release	Improved microvascular outcomes	Hypoglycemia; weight gain; may impede ischemic preconditioning
Meglitinides	1 to 2	Binds to sulfonylurea receptor, stimulating insulin release	Targets postprandial glucose; mimics physiological insulin secretion	Hypoglycemia; weight gain; frequent dosing
Thiazolidinediones	0.5 to 1.4	Increases peripheral insulin sensitivity	Potential β-cell preservation; no hypoglycemia	Edema, precipitating heart failure; weight gain
Alpha-glucosidase inhibitors	0.5 to 1	Retards gut carbohydrate absorption	Targets postprandial glucose; weight neutral	Intestinal gas; frequent dosing
GLP-1 agonist	0.5 to 1	Increases glucose-dependent insulin secretion	No hypoglycemia; weight loss	Nausea; vomiting; diarrhea
DPP-IV inhibitors	0.5	Block the degradation of GLP-1 and GIP, therefore increasing insulin	Weight neutral	Pancreatitis; skin reaction
Lipase inhibitors	None	Inhibit pancreatic and gastric lipases; blocks fat absorption	Weight loss	Diarrhea

Adapted from *Diabetes Facts and Guidelines 2009*. New Haven, CT: Yale Diabetes Center; 2009.

Table 1-4. Insulin Preparations and Pharmacokinetic Profile

Human Insulins and Analogues	Onset	Peaks (h)	Duration (h)
Rapid-acting			
Lispro/aspart	10 to 15 min	1 to 2	3 to 5
Regular	0.5 to 1 h	2 to 4	4 to 8
Intermediate-acting	1 to 4 h	4 to 12	10 to 20
Long-acting	2 to 3 h	None	24

Adapted from *Diabetes Facts and Guidelines 2009*. New Haven, CT: Yale Diabetes Center; 2009.

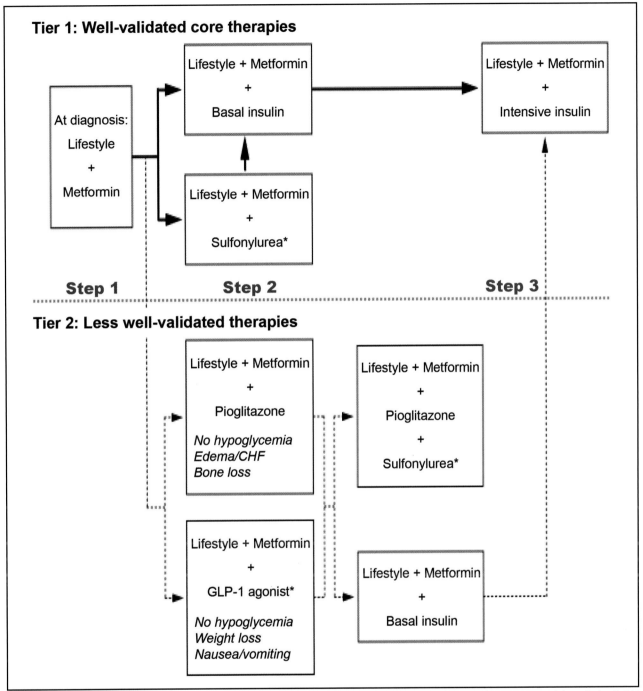

Figure 1-1. Algorithm for the metabolic management of type 2 diabetes; reinforce lifestyle interventions at every visit and check A1C every 3 months until A1C is <7% and then at least every 6 months. The interventions should be changed if A1C is ≥7 %.

REFERENCES

1. Expert Committee on the Diagnosis and Classification of Diabetes Mellitus. Report of the Expert Committee on the Diagnosis and Classification of Diabetes Mellitus. *Diabetes Care.* 1997;20:1183-1197.
2. American Diabetes Association. Diagnosis and classification of diabetes mellitus. *Diabetes Care.* 2009;32(Suppl 1):S62-S67.
3. Nabhan F, Emanuele MA, Emanuele N. Latent autoimmune diabetes of adulthood. Unique feature that distinguish it from types 1 and 2. *Postgrad Med.* 2005;117:7-12.
4. American Diabetes Association. Diagnosis and classification of diabetes mellitus. *Diabetes Care.* 2010;33(Suppl 1):S62-S69.
5. Expert Committee on the Diagnosis and Classification of Diabetes Mellitus. Follow-up report on the diagnosis of diabetes mellitus. *Diabetes Care.* 2003;26:3160-3167.
6. American Diabetes Association. Standards of medical care in diabetes—2009. *Diabetes Care.* 2009;32(Suppl 1):S13-S61.
7. International Expert Committee. International Expert Committee report on the role of the A1C assay in the diagnosis of diabetes. *Diabetes Care.* 2009;32:1327-1334.
8. Selvin E, Crainiceanu CM, Brancati FL, Coresh J. Short-term variability in measures of glycemia and implications for the classification of diabetes. *Arch Intern Med.* 2007;167:1545-1551.

9. Phillipou G, Phillips PJ. Intraindividual variation of glycohemoglobin: implications for interpretation and analytical goals. *Clin Chem.* 1993;39:2305-2308.

10. Rohlfing C, Wiedmeyer HM, Little R, et al. Biological variation of glycohemoglobin. *Clin Chem.* 2002;48:1116-1118.

11. Selvin E, Steffes M, Zhu H, et al. Glycated hemoglobin, diabetes, and cardiovascular risk in nondiabetic adults. *N Engl J Med.* 2010;362:800-811.

12. Chiasson JL, Aris-Jilwan N, Belanger R, et al. Diagnosis and treatment of diabetic ketoacidosis and the hyperglycemic hyperosmolar state. *CMAJ.* 2003;168:859-866.

13. Cryer PE. *Hypoglycemia in Diabetes. Pathophysiology, Prevalence and Prevention.* Alexandria, VA: American Diabetes Association; 2009.

14. Tight blood pressure control and risk of macrovascular and microvascular complications in type 2 diabetes: UKPDS 38. UK Prospective Diabetes Study Group. *BMJ.* 1998;317:703-713.

15. Arauz-Pacheco C, Parrott MA, Raskin P; American Diabetes Association. Hypertension management in adults with diabetes. *Diabetes Care.* 2004:27(Suppl 1):S65-S67.

16. Freeman R. Autonomic peripheral neuropathy. *Lancet.* 2005;365:1259-1270.

17. Sacco M, Pellegrini F, Roncaglioni MC, et al. Primary prevention of cardiovascular events with low-dose aspiring and vitamin E in type 2 diabetic patients: results of the Primary Prevention Project trial. *Diabetes Care.* 2003;26:3264-3272.

18. Hansson L, Zanchetti A, Carruthers SG, et al; HOT Study Group. Effects of intensive blood-pressure lowering and low-dose aspirin in patients with hypertension: principal results of the Hypertension Optimal Treatment (HOT) randomized trial. *Lancet.* 1998; 351:1755-1762.

19. Third Report of the National Cholesterol Education Program (NCEP) Expert Panel on Detection, Evaluation, and Treatment of High Blood Cholesterol in Adults (Adult Treatment Panel III) final report. *Circulation.* 2002;106:3143-3421.

20. Ford ES, Malarcher AM, Herman WH, Aubert RE. Diabetes mellitus and cigarette smoking: findings from the 1989 National Health Interview Survey. *Diabetes Care.* 1994;17:688-692.

21. Delamaire M, Maugendre M, Moreno M, et al. Impaired leukocyte functions in diabetic patients. *Diabet Med.* 1997;14:29-34.

22. Hostetter MK. Handicaps to host defense. Effects of hyperglycemia on C3 and Candida albicans. *Diabetes.* 1990;39:271-275.

23. Ferguson BJ. Mucormycosis of the nose and paranasal sinuses. *Otolaryngol Clin North Am.* 2000;33:349-365.

24. Nathan DM. Clinical practice. Initial management of glycemia in type 2 diabetes mellitus. *N Engl J Med.* 2002;347:1342-1349.

25. American Diabetes Association. *Medical Management of Type 2 Diabetes.* 6th ed. Alexandria, VA: American Diabetes Association; 2008.

26. Diabetes Control and Complications Trial Research Group. Progression of retinopathy with intensive versus conventional treatment in the Diabetes Control and Complications Trial. *Ophthalmology.* 1995;102:647-661.

27. American Diabetes Association. *Medical Management of Type 1 Diabetes.* 5th ed. Alexandria, VA: American Diabetes Association; 2008.

28. Knowler WC, Barrett-Connor E, Fowler SE, et al. Reduction in the incidence of type 2 diabetes with lifestyle intervention or metformin. *N Engl J Med.* 2002;346:393-403.

29. Bailey CJ, Turner RC. Metformin. *N Engl J Med.* 1996;334:574-579.

30. Hermann LS, Scherstén B, Bitzén PO, Kjellström T, Lindgärde F, Melander A. Therapeutic comparison of metformin and sulfonylurea, alone and in various combinations. A double blind controlled study. *Diabetes Care.* 1994;17:1100-1109.

31. Inzucchi SE. Oral antihyperglycemic therapy for type 2 diabetes: scientific review. *JAMA.* 2002;34:77-98.

32. Mellbin LG, Malmberg K, Norhammar A, Wedel H, Rydén L; DIGAMI 2 Investigators. Prognostic implications of glucose-lowering treatment in patients with acute myocardial infarction and diabetes: experiences from an extended follow-up of the Diabetes Mellitus Insulin-Glucose Infusion in Acute Myocardial Infarction (DIGAMI) 2 Study. *Diabetologia.* 2011;54(6):1308-1317.

33. The ADVANCE Collaborative Group. Intensive blood glucose control and vascular outcomes in patients with type 2 diabetes. *N Engl J Med.* 2008;358:2560-2572.

34. Intensive blood-glucose control with sulfonylureas or insulin compared with conventional treatment and risk of complications in patients with type 2 diabetes (UKPDS 33). UK Prospective Diabetes Study (UKPDS) Group. *Lancet.* 1998;352:837-853. Erratum in *Lancet.* 1999;354:602.

35. Nissen SE, Wolski K. Effect of rosiglitazone on the risk of myocardial infarction and death from cardiovascular causes. *N Engl J Med.* 2007;356:2457-2471. Erratum in *N Engl J Med.* 2007;357:100.

36. Schernthaner G, Matthews DR, Charbonnel B, et al. Efficacy and safety of pioglitazone versus metformin in patients with type 2 diabetes mellitus: a double-blind, randomized trial. *J Clin Endocrinol Metab.* 2004;89:6068-6076. Erratum in *J Clin Endocrinol Metab.* 2005;90:746.

37. Parkes DG, Pittner R, Jodka C, Smith P, Young A. Insulinotropic actions of exendin-4 and glucagon-like peptide-1 in vivo and in vitro. *Metabolism.* 2001;50:583-589.

38. Kolterman OG, Buse JB, Fineman MS, et al. Synthetic exendin-4 (exenatide) significantly reduces postprandial and fasting plasma glucose in subjects with type 2 diabetes. *J Clin Endocrinol Metab.* 2003;88:3082-3089.

39. DeFronzo RA, Ratner RE, Han J, et al. Effects of exenatide (exendin-4) on glycemic control and weight over 30 weeks in metformin-treated patients with type 2 diabetes. *Diabetes Care.* 2005;28:1092-1100.

40. Vilsboll T, Zdravkovic M, Le-Thi T, et al. Liraglutide, a long-acting human glucagon-like peptide-1 analog, given as monotherapy significantly improves glycemic control and lowers body weight without risk of hypoglycemia in patients with type 2 diabetes. *Diabetes Care.* 2007;30:1608-1610.

41. DeFronzo RA, Fleck PR, Wilson CA, Mekki Q. Efficacy and safety of the dipeptidyl peptidase-4 inhibitor alogliptin in patients with type 2 diabetes and inadequate glycemic control: a randomized, double-blind, placebo-controlled study. *Diabetes Care.* 2008; 31:2315-2317.

42. Chiasson JL, Josse RG, Hunt JA, et al. The efficacy of acarbose in the treatment of patients with non-insulin-dependent diabetes mellitus. A multicenter controlled clinical trial. *Ann Intern Med.* 1994;121:928-935.

43. Chiasson JL, Josse RG, Gomis R, Hanefeld M. Acarbose treatment and the risk of cardiovascular disease and hypertension in patients with impaired glucose tolerance: the STOP-NIDDM trial. *JAMA.* 2003;290:486-494.

44. Sjostrom L, Rissanen A, Andersen T, et al. Randomised placebo-controlled trial of orlistat for weight loss and prevention of weight regain in obese patients, European Multicentre Orlistat Study Group. *Lancet.* 1998;352:167-172.

45. Polonsky KS, Given BD, Van Cauter E. Twenty-four-hour profiles and pulsatile patterns of insulin secretion in normal and obese subjects. *J Clin Invest.* 1988;81:442-448.

46. Henry RR, Gumbiner B, Ditzler T, Wallace P, Lyon R, Glauber HS. Intensive conventional insulin therapy for type II diabetes: metabolic effects during a 6-mo outpatient trial. *Diabetes Care.* 1993;16:21-31.

47. *Diabetes Facts and Guidelines 2009.* New Haven, CT: Yale Diabetes Center; 2009.

2

Epidemiology and Pathogenesis of Diabetic Retinopathy

Susannah G. Rowe, MD, MPH and Alejandro Espaillat, MD

EPIDEMIOLOGY OF DIABETIC RETINOPATHY

Diabetes affects approximately 20 million people in the United States, and roughly 10 times that number worldwide.[1] The prevalence of diabetes has tripled in the United States over the past 25 years and has increased similarly rapidly throughout the rest of the world.[2] Experts foresee continued growth in the diabetic population, with projections that it will expand to include 439 million people by 2030.[3]

With the rapid increase in the prevalence of diabetics worldwide, the number of individuals at risk for diabetic retinopathy has increased dramatically in recent years. Diabetic retinopathy leads the list of microvascular complications of diabetes, affecting almost 90% of younger-onset (ie, in the first 3 decades of life) diabetics and over two-thirds of older-onset (ie, in the fourth decade and beyond) diabetics within 10 years after diagnosis.[4] Important risk factors for diabetic retinopathy include age, age of onset of diabetes, duration of diabetes, diabetes type and insulin use, and race/ethnicity. Systemic comorbidities play an important role, with hypertension, renal disease, dyslipidemias, elevated body mass index (BMI), and pregnancy all increasing the risk of developing retinopathy.

Age, Age of Onset, and Duration of Diabetes

At the time of diabetes diagnosis, between 6% and 34% of people show signs of diabetic retinopathy. Until approximately the seventh decade of life, these rates generally rise both with age and with increased time from diagnosis (Figure 2-1), although not in the same way for every type of diabetic.[2] Similarly, vision loss increases with age for every type of diabetes, although more so for older-onset diabetics, and less so for the oldest-old (ie, people in their 80s and older).

The amount of time elapsed since diagnosis of diabetes predicts the prevalence of both nonproliferative and proliferative diabetic retinopathy among patients taking insulin.[4] Among patients taking insulin for diabetes diagnosed at a younger age, the incidence of diabetic retinopathy and proliferative diabetic retinopathy rises over the first 10 years after diagnosis. The 25-year cumulative risk of developing diabetic retinopathy in this group is high, with reports ranging from 89% to 97%.[5,6] However, after 20 or more years, the diabetic retinopathy rate of progression in this group tends to slow, and the severity of diabetic retinopathy tends to improve over time. Among insulin-taking diabetics who were diagnosed at an older age, the rate of incidence and progression of diabetic retinopathy also declines over time. Older-onset diabetics who do not take insulin show a very different pattern. In this group, time from

Espaillat A.
Diabetic Eye Disease: A Comprehensive Review (pp. 11-14)
© 2012 SLACK Incorporated

Figure 2-1. Prevalence of diabetic retinopathy by age in different populations.

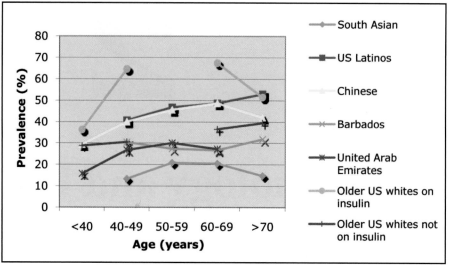

diagnosis of diabetes has little predictive value in terms of incidence of new retinopathy or progression of diabetic retinopathy.

In the oldest-old age range, patients in some studies show a decrease in prevalence and severity of retinopathy, possibly related to decreased survival of sicker patients over time. In general, type 1 diabetics who are diagnosed before their 30s are somewhat more likely to develop diabetic retinopathy than those diagnosed later in life.[4]

There is some suggestion that continued improvements in diagnosis and control of risk factors have reduced the burden of diabetic retinopathy. In 25-year data from the Wisconsin Epidemiologic Study of Diabetic Retinopathy (WESDR), younger-onset diabetics who have been diagnosed more recently appear to be doing better in terms of nonproliferative diabetic retinopathy than those diagnosed at the same age decades ago.[6] These data further suggest that more timely diagnosis and intervention for diabetic retinopathy have reduced the incidence of visual impairment in this population.[7]

Diabetes Type and Insulin Use

As previously noted, the type of diabetes greatly influences the course of diabetic retinopathy. Type I diabetics are much less likely to shows signs of diabetic retinopathy at diagnosis than type 2 diabetics. On initial ophthalmic examination following diagnosis of diabetes, type I diabetics have reported retinopathy prevalence rates of 0% to 3% as opposed to 7% to 38% for type 2 diabetics.[1,2,8] However, the 25-year WESDR data suggest that prevalence rates for the 2 types of diabetes do not vary after adjusting for duration of diabetes. This finding may be consistent with other studies that have found onset of type 2 diabetes can be difficult to pinpoint precisely.

Race/Ethnicity

Reports suggest that the incidence and prevalence of diabetic retinopathy may vary by race/ethnicity (see Figure 2-1). Hispanic Caucasian populations lead with the highest reported prevalence, with 46% of type 2 diabetics in one study showing signs of diabetic retinopathy.[9] Almost 34% of Latino diabetics progress to diabetic retinopathy after 4 years.[10]

Studies comparing the severity of diabetic retinopathy in non-Hispanic Blacks versus non-Hispanic Whites do not offer consistent results. Other studies comparing incidence and prevalence rates have suggested that differences in quality of care and social factors may confound any biologic differences that exist.[2]

SYSTEMIC COMORBIDITIES

Hypertension, renal disease, dyslipidemia, and elevated BMI are all significant risk factors for diabetic retinopathy. Dose-response curves demonstrate worsening diabetic retinopathy with greater severity of these comorbid conditions. Furthermore, control of these conditions leads to improved outcomes of diabetic retinopathy. Pregnancy represents an independent risk factor for diabetes.

Diabetic Retinopathy Without Diabetes

Numerous reports describe a population of patients who have retinal changes that meet criteria for diabetic retinopathy but whose serum glucose measurements do not meet criteria for diabetes mellitus.[2] Hypertension, elevated BMI, advanced age, and diagnosis via photography versus clinical examination are all associated with these findings.

Diabetes Without Diabetic Retinopathy

The 50-Year Medalist Study[11] describes a cross-sectional survey of 326 individuals who have been living with type 1 diabetes for 50 or more years. Despite the extreme duration of diabetes in this group, many of these individuals appear to be relatively resistant to the microvascular complications of the disease. In fact, approximately 40% of the individuals in this study remained free of significant diabetic retinopathy 50 to 80 years after onset of diabetes. Furthermore, a number of the usual risk factors for microvascular disease do not appear to apply. In fact, age, diabetes duration, age at onset of diabetes, HbA1C, BMI, total cholesterol, and LDL cholesterol did not significantly predict the likelihood of suffering retinal complications of diabetes. These individuals did far better if they exercised more or if they had higher HDL levels (although these 2 protective factors were not additive). Research from the Medalist Study has shown that based on laboratory studies, many of these patients appear to have a variant of type 1 diabetes while retaining some evidence of insulin production.[11]

Pathophysiology of Diabetic Retinopathy

Nonproliferative Diabetic Retinopathy

Diabetes affects every major cell type in the retina, including neurons, glial and microglial cells, vascular cells, and pigment epithelial cells.[12] Initially, activation of many of these cell types occurs. Activation alters the production of mediators, such as growth and coagulation factors, and modifies cell-to-cell interactions. Clinically, loss of neuroretinal function represents one of the earliest detectable signs of diabetic retinopathy.[13]

Early in the disease process, autoregulation of blood flow fails, and blood flow through the retinal vasculature increases. Arterioles and venules lengthen and dilate. Deregulation of cell turnover, apoptosis, and oxidative stress result in loss of pericytes. Capillaries become increasingly permeable as the blood-retinal barrier breaks down and intraretinal hemorrhages and edema become apparent. Basement membranes thicken and the extracellular matrix proliferates. Inflammatory and pro-coagulant factors slow blood flow through already damaged capillaries, resulting in loss of smaller vessels and further oxidative stress.

Proliferative Diabetic Retinopathy

Although the explosion of knowledge regarding mechanisms of normal and abnormal angiogenesis in the retina has greatly enriched the current understanding of the pathogenesis of proliferative diabetic retinopathy, a great deal of debate remains regarding the exact mechanisms underlying these pathologic processes. General consensus exists that proliferative diabetic retinopathy ensues when hyperglycemia persists for too long at levels that are toxic to the retina. Capillary nonperfusion and cell death or apoptosis, mediated by tumor necrosis factor-a (TNF-α) and other factors, result in acellular capillaries that do not perfuse adjacent retinal tissue. Nonperfusion leads to hypoxia of the inner retinal layers and associated reactions to oxidative stress. As a direct consequence of the resultant hypoxic insult, researchers noted increases in a complex series of growth factors, including hypoxia-inducible factor-1a (HIF-1), growth hormone (GH), insulin-like growth factor 1 (IGF-1), hepatocyte growth factor (HGF), platelet-derived growth factor (PDGF), basic fibroblast growth factor (b-FGF), angiopoietins, integrins, proinflammatory cytokines, and other factors.[1,14]

Anti-angiogenic influences such as somatostatin are simultaneously quelled. The normal balance of angiogenic and anti-angiogenic factors degenerates.[15] Vascular remodeling and new blood vessel growth, or neovascularization, ensue.

Underlying Mechanisms of Diabetic Retinopathy

Experts agree that diabetic retinopathy originates with hyperglycemia. Abundant evidence demonstrates that elevated glucose levels in the retina initiate a complex series of responses, some independent and some interrelated, that ultimately lead to the characteristic microvascular changes seen in the diabetic retina. Several major lines of research have attempted to elucidate the connection between hyperglycemia and microvascular damage. These include increased polyol pathway flux, advanced glycation end-products (AGEs), activation of protein kinase C (PKC), increased hexosamine pathway flux, and activation of the renin-angiotensin system. The unified theory of diabetic retinopathy postulates that many of these pathways ultimately lead to increased oxidative stress due to the formation of reactive oxygen species (ROS).[2] Increasing evidence highlights the contribution of neurodegeneration and inflammation, as well as angiogenesis, in the pathogenesis of diabetic retinopathy.

Polyol Pathway Flux

Activation of the polyol pathway occurs in diabetes. When glucose levels are high, aldose reductase processes excess glucose to sorbitol via this pathway. Nicotinamide adenine dinucleotide phosphate (NADPH) functions as a cofactor in this process. As NADPH is consumed processing glucose to sorbitol, it therefore becomes less available to regenerate reduced glutathione. NADPH eventually reconstitutes as sorbitol, and ultimately converts to fructose. However, its reduced availability to regenerate glutathione has been postulated as a contributor to oxidative stress.

Advanced Glycation End-Products

AGEs develop under hyperglycemic conditions, generated from early glycation end products that result from altered glucose metabolism. Elevated levels of AGEs interfere with multiple processes within the retina. An increase in AGEs in diabetic blood vessels alters extracellular matrix components, and integrins, disrupting matrix-cell interactions. AGEs also decrease the number of healthy pericytes, promoting capillary permeability and blood-retinal barrier breakdown. Researchers note an increase in receptor-mediated production of ROS associated with elevated levels of AGEs.

Activation of Protein Kinase C

Hyperglycemia indirectly activates many of PKC's 11 isoforms throughout retinal tissues. The complex cascade of reactions to elevated PKC involves alterations in cellular signaling, transduction, and increases in vascular endothelial growth factor. Vascular changes include perturbations in blood flow, leukocyte vascular adhesion, and vascular permeability. Increased extracellular matrix protein expansion results from synthesis of type IV collagen, TGF-b1, and fibronectin.

Increased Hexosamine Pathway Flux

Increased flux through the hexosamine pathway occurs when intracellular glucose levels are high. Activation of this pathway results in altered gene activation and modifications in gene transcription that are associated with vascular endothelial dysfunction.

Activation of the Renin-Angiotensin System

Angiotensin affects vascular smooth muscle cells and the accumulation of extracellular matrix proteins. The activated renin-angiotensin system in diabetes has received extensive attention as an important pathway in microvascular damage. In fact, inhibition of the renin-angiotensin system can delay onset of early retinopathy, although it has little effect on progression of retinopathy in the more advanced stages.[16]

Inflammation

Inflammatory mediators, including proinflammatory cytokines and chemokines, lead to chronic, low-grade inflammation in the diabetic retina. Leukocytes drawn to the retina accumulate, and elevated levels of factors such as TNF-α increase leukocyte–endothelial cell adhesion. The resultant leukostasis worsens capillary nonperfusion and endothelial cell damage. Several investigations have demonstrated upregulation of cyclooxygenase-2 in diabetic tissues; these findings may help delineate the mechanisms underlying chronic inflammation and microvascular damage in diabetes.

REFERENCES

1. Williams R, Airey M, Baxter H, et al. Epidemiology of diabetic retinopathy and macular oedema: a systematic review. *Eye.* 2004;18:963-983.
2. Bhavsar AR, Emerson GG, Emerson MV, Browning DJ. Epidemiology of diabetic retinopathy. In: Browning DJ, ed. *Diabetic Retinopathy Evidence-Based Management.* New York, NY: Springer; 2010:53-75.
3. Wild S, Roglic G, Green A, et al. Global prevalence of diabetes: estimates for the year 2000 and projections for 2030. *Diabetes Care.* 2004;27:1047-1053.
4. Klein R, Klein B, Moss S, Cruickshanks K. The Wisconsin epidemiologic study of diabetic retinopathy. *Arch Ophthalmol.* 1994;112:1217-1228.
5. Skrivarhaug T, Fosmark DS, Stene LC, et al. Low cumulative incidence of proliferative diabetic retinopathy in childhood-onset type 1 diabetes: a 24-year follow-up study. *Diabetologia.* 2006;49:2281-2290.
6. Klein R, Lee KE, Gangnon RE, Klein BE. The 25-year incidence of visual impairment in type 1 diabetes mellitus the Wisconsin epidemiologic study of diabetic retinopathy. *Ophthalmology.* 2010;117:63-70.
7. Klein R, Lee KE, Knudtson MD, Gangnon RE, Klein BE. Changes in visual impairment prevalence by period of diagnosis of diabetes: the Wisconsin Epidemiologic Study of Diabetic Retinopathy. *Ophthalmology.* 2009;116:1937-1942.
8. Al-Maskari F, El-Sadig M. Prevalence of diabetic retinopathy in the United Arab Emirates: a cross-sectional survey. *BMC Ophthalmol.* 2007;7:11-19.
9. Varma R, Torres M, Peña F, Klein R, Azen SP; Los Angeles Latino Eye Study Group. Prevalence of diabetic retinopathy in adult Latinos: the Los Angeles Latino eye study. *Ophthalmology.* 2004;111:1298-1306.
10. Varma R, Choudhury F, Klein R, Chung J, Torres M, Azen SP; Los Angeles Latino Eye Study Group. Four-year incidence and progression of diabetic retinopathy and macular edema: the Los Angeles Latino Eye Study. *Am J Ophthalmol.* 2010;149:752-761.
11. Keenan HA, Costacou T, Sun JK, et al. Clinical factors associated with resistance to microvascular complications in diabetic patients of extreme disease duration: the 50-Year Medalist Study. *Diabetes Care.* 2007;30:1995-1997.
12. El-Asrar AMA, Al-Mezaine HS, Ola MS. Pathophysiology and management of diabetic retinopathy. *Expert Rev Ophthalmol.* 2009;4:627-646.
13. Antonetti DA, Barber AJ, Bronson SK, et al. Diabetic retinopathy: seeing beyond glucose-induced microvascular disease. *Diabetes.* 2006;55:2401-2411.
14. Stewart MW. Pathophysiology of diabetic retinopathy. In: Browning DJ, ed. *Diabetic Retinopathy Evidence-Based Management.* New York, NY: Springer; 2010:1-30.
15. Simo R, Carrasco E, Garcia-Ramirez M, Hernandez C. Angiogenic and antiangiogenic factors in proliferative diabetic retinopathy. *Curr Diabetes Rev.* 2006;2:71-98.
16. Perkins BA, Aiello LP, Krolewski AS. Diabetes complications and the renin–angiotensin system. *N Engl J Med.* 2009;361:83-85.

3

Diabetes Mellitus and Cranial Neuropathies of the Eye and Orbit

Deval (Reshma) Paranjpe, MD and Alejandro Espaillat, MD

Diabetic microvascular ischemic disease can affect both peripheral nerves and cranial nerves (CNs). Diabetes is a major risk factor for cranial ocular motor nerve palsies, and diabetics have been reported to have a 7.5-fold greater incidence of ischemic ocular motor nerve palsies.[1] Ischemic palsies of CNs III, IV, and VI result in diplopia, ocular misalignment, and patient discomfort.[2] Although diabetic ischemic disease is a recognized and common cause of each of these palsies, it is critical to rule out life-threatening etiologies such as aneurysm, tumor, and infection, particularly fungal infection.[3]

Other CNs can also be affected by diabetes. CN II, the optic nerve, can be affected by nerve fiber dropout and papillitis, and optic neuropathy can occur in young diabetics.[4] Dialysis-related optic neuropathy has also been described.[5] Diabetic peripheral neuropathy can affect CN V, causing trigeminal neuralgia.[6] Finally, CN VII can be affected, producing a scenario mimicking Bell's palsy.[7] Multiple studies have correlated lack of glycemic control to incidence of cranial neuropathies in diabetics, although some studies have failed to show any direct link.[8]

PALSIES OF CRANIAL NERVES III, IV, AND VI

Third, fourth, and sixth CN palsies are the most commonly found among diabetic patients.[2] Most often, these palsies are found in isolation, but occasionally they may be found in conjunction. The cavernous sinus is a likely locale for pathology as multiple CNs pass through it and can be simultaneously affected by thrombosis; tumor; and infiltrative, vascular, or other lesions. Similarly, the brainstem can also be a location for pathology involving multiple CNs at their origins.[9]

Apart from the usual concern of brainstem lesion or cavernous sinus tumor, infection is a serious concern in diabetics, especially in those with poor glycemic control. Single or multiple cranial motor nerve palsies can be the sentinel sign of an advancing infectious process in diabetics.[9] Fungal infections such as aspergillosis and mucormycosis can originate in the sinus cavities and spread to surrounding tissues in diabetics, typically in those with poor glycemic control or other immunocompromising factors.[9] These infections must be detected quickly and treated aggressively and often surgically if the patient is to survive.

Espaillat A.
Diabetic Eye Disease: A Comprehensive Review (pp. 15-20)
© 2012 SLACK Incorporated

Pain in Microvascular Ischemic Ocular Motor Cranial Nerve Palsies

Pain is a common feature of ischemic microvascular CN palsies regardless of the presence of diabetes in the patient. A recent study of 87 patients with acute onset of cranial ocular motor nerve palsies showed that most such palsies are painful, with the pain either preceding or accompanying the onset of diplopia.[10] Diabetics experience similar characteristics and rates of pain as nondiabetics. Pain is typically experienced in the ipsilateral eye and brow, and duration of pain is longer with increased severity of pain, with severe pain lasting approximately 1 month whereas mild to moderate pain resolves.[10]

Third Cranial Nerve Palsy

Any patient presenting with a third nerve palsy should be evaluated emergently as the most serious cause (ie, aneurysm involving the junction of the posterior communicating and internal carotid arteries) can be rapidly fatal. More than one neuro-ophthalmologist has related the story of a patient referred with a third nerve palsy who collapsed from ruptured intracranial aneurysm before his or her eyes. Another serious but less immediately fatal cause of third nerve palsy is tumor compressing the third nerve along its course. Therefore, a third nerve palsy must never be ascribed to microvascular cause and dismissed as a "diabetic third nerve palsy" without thorough examination.[3]

A complete third nerve palsy consists of complete ipsilateral ptosis and complete paralysis of ipsilateral elevation, depression, and adduction.[2] An incomplete third nerve palsy refers to varying degrees of the above signs. Pupillary involvement denotes any amount of dilation of the ipsilateral pupil relative to the other side, with significant involvement resulting in the "blown pupil." A pupil-involving third nerve palsy must be treated as a potentially life-threatening emergency.[2]

Lee and Brazis distinguish 6 major types of third CN palsies. Type 1 is nonisolated, comprising severe headache, orbital or myasthenic signs, multiple CN involvement, brainstem signs, associated temporal arteritis, collagen vascular disease, or cancer. Type 2 is isolated and traumatic in origin. Type 3 is congenital. Type 4 is isolated, acquired, and nontraumatic (types 4a and 4b represent normal pupillary function with complete or incomplete extraocular muscle palsies, respectively; type 4c represents subnormal pupillary function with any degree of extraocular muscle function). Type 5 is a progressive or unresolved third nerve palsy. Type 6 features aberrant regeneration of the nerve.[11]

Type 4a is most commonly ischemic in origin and strongly associated with the presence of diabetes mellitus.[3] Other entities that should be considered in the differential diagnosis of diabetic microvascular CN palsy include temporal arteritis, systemic lupus erythematosus, and use of sildenafil citrate or cocaine.[3,12,13]

Anatomy

The fibers of the third CN split into 2 divisions only after passing into the orbit through the superior orbital fissure. The superior division innervates the superior rectus and levator muscle, thus controlling supraduction and lid elevation. The inferior division innervates the pupillary constrictor muscle, medial and inferior recti, and inferior oblique.[12] If functions of both branches of the nerve are affected, the lesion affects the preorbital portion of the nerve; if only one branch is affected, the lesion usually is within the orbit.[12] However, divisional or focal third nerve palsies that are pupil sparing should be examined carefully for aneurysmal involvement. Nerve fibers from the Edinger-Westphal nucleus that innervate the pupillary constrictor run peripherally within the third nerve in the area of the junction of the posterior communicating and internal carotid arteries. Therefore, a compressive lesion (typically an aneurysm or tumor) impinging upon the third nerve in this area will directly affect these peripheral pupillary fibers and result in dilation of the ipsilateral pupil.[12] Ischemic lesions, in contrast, affect the central fibers of the third nerve rather than the peripheral region and thus tend not to affect the pupillary fibers.[13]

Documented locations for diabetic microvascular third nerve lesions in postmortem studies include the cavernous sinus and subarachnoid portions, and although mesencephalic lesions have been shown, most lesions tend to be peripheral. Pain in diabetic microvascular palsies may result from ischemic damage to first-division trigeminal fibers carried either in the connective tissue sheath of the third CN within the cavernous sinus or within the oculomotor nerve or trochlear nerves, as shown in animal studies.

Symptoms

Symptoms of third CN palsies include binocular diplopia, ipsilateral ptosis, anisocoria (in pupil-involving palsies), and pain. Patients with third nerve palsies present most commonly with binocular diplopia with images often separated diagonally. Diplopia may not be noticed by the patient if significant ipsilateral ptosis is also present, or if visual acuity in either eye is impaired. Ipsilateral ptosis ranges in severity and will be complete in a complete third nerve palsy.[12]

Pupil-involving palsies will present with a dilated ipsilateral pupil, and the patient or accompanying family/friends may point out the noticeable anisocoria. Pain may or may not be present with any type of third nerve palsy and should not be used as a diagnostic criterion to determine etiology. Classically, aneurysmal palsies are more apt to be painful whereas diabetic/microvascular palsies tend to be painless; however, the reverse can also be true.[10]

Signs

The eye in complete third nerve palsy will have complete paralysis of adductor, elevator, and depressor function and will therefore be exotropic (due to unopposed CN VI function) and hypotropic/slightly intorted compared to the normal eye in direct gaze (due to unopposed CN IV function).[2]

Ptosis

Complete third nerve palsy produces complete ipsilateral ptosis; incomplete palsies produce incomplete ptosis.[2]

Involvement of the Pupil

As mentioned above, ipsilateral pupillary dilation should be treated as an emergency due to possible risk of impending aneurysmal rupture.[3] Diabetic third nerve palsies are typically not associated with pupillary involvement; however, trace anisocoria up to 1 mm can be observed, although rare.[3] This is a matter of purely esoteric interest, however. In practice, any degree of pupillary involvement in a complete or incomplete third nerve palsy, no matter how slight, should be treated as a potential aneurysmal risk and the patient should be transported to the emergency department immediately. Many authors recommend noninvasive studies such as magnetic resonance imaging/magnetic resonance angiogram (MRI/MRA) or computed tomography (CT) angiography for all patients with third nerve palsy regardless of circumstances, except for patients with complete third nerve palsy with a normal pupil.[3,11]

Disposition and Workup

- *Pupil-involving third nerve palsy in any patient of any age or disease state*: Immediate transport to hospital, emergent neuroimaging to exclude aneurysm/other compressive lesion. This may include MRI with and without contrast, MRA, or CT or conventional angiography, which has been the gold standard historically.
- *Pupil-sparing incomplete third nerve palsy in any age group or disease state*: The physician should obtain a noninvasive neuroimaging (MRI/MRA or CT angiography) immediately, to eliminate the possibility of compressive lesion. If these diagnostic tests are not available, the physician must follow-up with the patient daily to monitor for any development of pupillary involvement.

- *Pupil-sparing complete third nerve palsy in a patient older than 55 years, diabetic or potential vasculopaths*: The patient should be followed to ensure no pupillary involvement or other cranial neuropathy develops; urgent imaging is not indicated as the cause is likely microvascular. Sedimentation rate (ESR) should be checked to rule out temporal arteritis; a workup for diabetes, hypertension, vasculitis, sarcoidosis, or other cause for microvascular disease is indicated, if not already known. Many patients will have progression of palsy symptoms, with peak at 10 days after onset. Resolution is expected between 1 and 3 months; during this time, patching may help with diplopia. Neuroimaging should be performed if the palsy does not resolve in 12 weeks.
- *Pupil-sparing complete nerve palsy in nonvasculopathic patient without risk factors listed above*: Neuroimaging (MRI/MRA) is indicated.

Special Cases

Aberrant Regeneration of Third Nerve

Aberrant regeneration is rarely ever seen in microvascular disease and signs thereof should not be ascribed to diabetic third nerve palsy. Instead, a compressive mass lesion (usually in the cavernous sinus) should be sought; these lesions usually are slow growing, as the nerve fibers have had time to aberrantly regenerate after initial insult, often months to years afterward. Signs of aberrant regeneration of the third CN include adduction on elevation or depression; lid retraction with downgaze or adduction; or pupillary miosis on upgaze, downgaze, or adduction.[14]

Myasthenia Gravis

Myasthenia gravis, which affects the neuromuscular junction, can produce muscular effects resembling a painless third nerve palsy (pupil sparing), or for that matter, any CN palsy. To distinguish this condition from a microvascular palsy, look for weakness of the orbicularis oculi, no ptosis/diplopia on waking with subsequent progression during the day, and increased ptosis of either upper eyelid when the opposite eyelid is manually elevated. An ice or Tensilon test is diagnostic, and neuro-ophthalmic/neurology referral is indicated.[15,16]

Testing for Associated Fourth Cranial Nerve Palsy

In third nerve palsy, the eye will still intort in downgaze if fourth nerve function is preserved. If intorsion on downgaze is absent, both a third and fourth CN palsy are present. Tumor, infiltrative, or infectious causes should be considered with likely location being the cavernous sinus.[2]

Fourth Cranial Nerve Palsy

Urgency

An ophthalmologic evaluation should be conducted within 1 week.

Anatomy and Function

The trochlear or fourth CN innervates the superior oblique muscle and thus functions to intort and depress the eye. It travels in close proximity to the third and fifth CNs in the cavernous sinus area before entering the orbit through the superior orbital fissure to innervate the superior oblique. Congenital palsies are common and are the most common cause of fourth nerve palsy in children.[11]

Lee and Brazis categorize fourth nerve palsies into 6 types.[11] Type 1 is nonisolated, with other neurologic or systemic associations. Type 2 is traumatic with an obvious history of head trauma. Type 3 is congenital. Type 4 is vasculopathic; it is found in either patients aged >50 years possibly with hypertension and/or diabetes, or younger patients who are known vasculopaths. Type 5 is nonvasculopathic and does not qualify for any of the previous categories. Type 6 is progressive or unresolved; these entail either worsening after the first week of onset or failure of the measured deviation to improve after 6 to 8 weeks.

Signs and Symptoms

The Bielschowsky 3-step test will be positive. Ipsilateral hypertropia and excyclotorsion occurs in fourth nerve palsy and will be greater with contralateral gaze and ipsilateral head tilt. The patient unconsciously tilts his head away from the side of the palsy to relieve symptoms. In congenital palsy cases, this can be elicited from photographs dating back to childhood, which will show a characteristic head tilt. Although trauma is the leading cause of CN IV palsy in adults, 5% to 10% of these palsies are caused by diabetic microvascular disease. Other causes may include hypertension and atherosclerosis.[13]

The differential diagnosis of diabetic microvascular fourth nerve palsy should also include myasthenia gravis, temporal arteritis, inferior rectus entrapment in the setting of trauma, thyroid eye disease, infection, tumor, cavernous sinus lesion, skew deviation (especially when seen with brainstem/cerebellar symptoms), and demyelinating disease.[13]

Evaluation

Blood work for temporal arteritis (ESR), myasthenia autoantibody panel, fasting blood glucose, complete blood count, and thyroid panel can be obtained as indicated by symptoms. Diabetic and hypertensive workups should be conducted in patients without obvious risk factors, as several studies have shown that an isolated nerve palsy can be a presenting symptom of microvascular disease.[2] CT of the orbits with coronal and axial cuts should be performed if trauma is a consideration. MRI of the brain and orbits should be performed to rule out a structural lesion such as tumor impacting fourth nerve, especially in type 1, 5, and 6 palsies.

Diabetic fourth nerve palsies usually do not require immediate neuroimaging studies and can be observed for 6 to 8 weeks. Spontaneous resolution can be expected within 6 months in most cases; no resolution within 2 months may trigger consideration of MRI.

Disposition and Treatment

Patching, frosting, or covering the spectacle lens of the affected eye may be needed initially to alleviate patient distress. If the palsy is diabetic, it should slowly resolve over several months and Fresnel prisms (temporary adhesive prisms applied to the back surface of the patient's spectacle lens) can reduce or eliminate diplopia. As the palsy improves, the patient can be "weaned" to less powerful Fresnel prisms until none are needed to correct the diplopia. Prisms can also be permanently ground into the spectacle lens in the case of longstanding palsies where Fresnel correction has worked; however, this can be expensive. If the palsy has not resolved, imaging is normal and the extent of deviation has been stable for at least 6 months, extraocular muscle surgery may be considered for relief of the diplopia.

Sixth Cranial Nerve Palsy

A common cause of sixth CN palsy in older patients is diabetic or hypertensive microvascular ischemia. Other causes include compression from tumor or aneurysm, trauma, and inflammation. Increased intracranial pressure (caused by pseudotumor cerebri or mass lesion) may also cause sixth nerve palsy via a compressive effect. Brainstem lesions involving the sixth nerve nucleus may also affect the seventh nerve and cause internuclear ophthalmoplegia, gaze palsy, or Horner syndrome. The sixth CN courses through the cavernous sinus and may be affected by pathology therein along with other CNs.[17]

Lee and Brazis classify 6 types of sixth CN palsy. Type 1 is nonisolated and occurs with other brainstem or systemic symptoms. Type 2 is post-traumatic. Type 3 is congenital. Type 4 is vasculopathic, occurring in patients aged >55 years or who have diabetes, hypertension, or other vasculopathic conditions. Type 5 is nonvasculopathic but does not qualify in any of the previous categories. Type 6 is progressive or nonresolving sixth nerve palsy.[11]

Symptoms

Horizontal binocular diplopia and pain (even in diabetic/microvascular sixth nerve palsies).

Signs

Ipsilateral esotropia. Check for papilledema to rule out increased intracranial pressure as a cause.

Differential Diagnosis of Relatively Acute Onset Nontraumatic Sixth Nerve Palsy

Among the possible causes of a relative acute onset nontraumatic sixth nerve palsy are thyroid eye disease, orbital pseudotumor, myasthenia gravis, temporal arteritis, multiple sclerosis, aneurysm, vasculopathic, and orbital cellulitis.

Workup

Microvascular palsy and idiopathic palsies should, while common, essentially be diagnoses of exclusion in patients without known vasculopathy. Mass lesions and cavernous sinus processes should be excluded using MRI; if papilledema is present and no mass lesion is present on MRI, lumbar puncture should be performed. Patients with post-traumatic palsies from a closed head injury would typically have been imaged at the time of the initial injury. Neurological and neurosurgical consultation should be obtained as appropriate to clinical findings.

Disposition

Diabetic, other microvascular, idiopathic, and traumatic palsies spontaneously resolve over time, typically by 3 months. As with other palsies causing diplopia, patching may help with comfort while improvement occurs. Botulinum toxin in the medial rectus muscle may help bring the eye back to neutral position in primary gaze, and in chronic sixth nerve palsy without improvement, surgical correction may be attempted.

OTHER DIABETIC CRANIAL NEUROPATHIES OF OPHTHALMIC INTEREST

Optic Nerve: Nerve Fiber Layer Dropout

Mean retinal nerve fiber layer thickness has been shown to be significantly less in diabetics with normal microvasculature than in nondiabetic individuals, resulting in a corresponding decrease in fibers in the optic nerve. Low nerve fiber layer thickness in patients with preclinical diabetic retinopathy is mildly associated with poorer glycemic control.[18,19]

Wolfram Syndrome

Wolfram syndrome or DIDMOAD (diabetes insipidus, diabetes mellitus, optic atrophy, and deafness) is a progressive, neurodegenerative disorder with an autosomal recessive inheritance pattern and onset in early childhood. One in 150 children with juvenile insulin-dependent diabetes mellitus will have DIDMOAD. Any child with well-controlled diabetes mellitus exhibiting polyuria and polydipsia, hearing loss, or unexplained visual loss should be evaluated for optic atrophy and DIDMOAD. Death usually occurs before age 50 and quality of life is poor due to serious morbidities associated with various facets of the DIDMOAD syndrome.[20,21]

Dialysis-Related Optic Neuropathy

End-stage renal disease due to diabetic complications results in patients dependent on dialysis for survival. Repeated or prolonged episodes of hypotensive ischemia during dialysis can result in bilateral, permanent visual loss due to anterior ischemic optic neuropathy. Anemia, which is also frequently found in dialysis-dependent patients, can aggravate this situation.[22]

TRIGEMINAL NERVE

Fibers of the first division of the trigeminal nerve are associated with the connective tissue sheath of the third CN within the cavernous sinus and therefore can be affected by any of the pathologic processes causing third nerve palsy. In addition, animal studies have shown that first division trigeminal fibers can be found within the third and fourth CNs and can be thus affected. The trigeminal nerve can also be involved in isolation as a focal painful peripheral diabetic neuropathy.[23]

FACIAL NERVE

Peripheral facial palsy seems to be a focal neuropathic involvement rather than part of a multifocal involvement pattern in diabetics. Although severity was similar between diabetics and nondiabetics within the first month of onset, diabetics have a significantly slower rate of recovery from facial nerve palsy than nondiabetic counterparts. Histopathologic studies of the human temporal bone and facial nerve canal in diabetics and nondiabetics reveal ischemia of the facial nerve in diabetics compared to controls. This is thought to be the basis of slower recovery from palsy in diabetic patients.[24]

REFERENCES

1. Wilker SC, Rucker JC, Newman NJ, Biousse V, Tomsak RL. Pain in ischaemic ocular motor cranial nerve palsies. *Br J Ophthalmol.* 2009;93:1657-1659.

2. Brazis PW. Isolated palsies of cranial nerves III, IV, and VI. *Semin Neurol.* 2009;29:14-28.

3. Jacobson DM. Pupil involvement in patients with diabetes-associated oculomotor nerve palsy. *Arch Ophthalmol.* 1998;116:723-727.

4. Hayreh SS, Zimmerman MB. Nonarteritic anterior ischemic optic neuropathy: clinical characteristics in diabetic patients versus nondiabetic patients. *Ophthalmology.* 2008;115:1818-1825.

5. Basile C, Addabbo G, Montanaro A. Anterior ischemic optic neuropathy and dialysis: role of hypotension and anemia. *J Nephrol.* 2001;14:420-423.

6. Takayama S, Osawa M, Takahashi Y, Iwamoto Y. Painful neuropathy with trigeminal nerve involvement in type 2 diabetes. *J Int Med Res.* 2006;34:115-118.

7. Kariya S, Cureoglu S, Morita N, et al. Vascular findings in the facial nerve canal in human temporal bones with diabetes mellitus. *Otol Neurotol.* 2009;30(3):402-407.

8. Singh NP, Garg S, Kumar S, Gulati S. Multiple cranial nerve palsies associated with type 2 diabetes mellitus. *Singapore Med J.* 2006;47:712-715.

9. Eshbaugh CG, Siatkowski RM, Smith JL, Kline LB. Simultaneous, multiple cranial neuropathies in diabetes mellitus. *J Neuroophthalmol.* 1995;15:219-224.

10. Bortolami R, D'Alessandro R, Manni E. The origin of pain in ischemic-diabetic third-nerve palsy. *Arch Neurol.* 1993;50:795.

11. Lee AG, Brazis PW. *Clinical Pathways in Neuro-Ophthalmology: An Evidence-Based Approach.* 2nd ed. New York, NY: Thieme; 2003.

12. Levin LA, Arnold AC. *Neuro-Ophthalmology: The Practical Guide.* New York, NY: Thieme; 2005.

13. Watanabe K, Hagura R, Akanuma Y, et al. Characteristics of cranial nerve palsies in diabetic patients. *Diabetes Res Clin Pract.* 1990;10:19-27.

14. Kiziltan ME, Akalin MA, Sahin R, Uluduz D. Peripheral neuropathy in patients with diabetes mellitus presenting as Bell's palsy. *Neurosci Lett.* 2007;427:138-141.

15. Said G. Diabetic neuropathy—a review. *Nat Clin Pract Neurol.* 2007;3:331-340.

16. Said G. Diabetic neuropathy: an update. *J Neurol.* 1996;243:431-440.

17. Choplin NT. Diabetes-associated retinal nerve fiber damage evaluated with scanning laser polarimetry. *Am J Ophthalmol.* 2006;142:88-94.

18. Gupta PK, Bhatti MT, Rucker JC. A sweet case of bilateral sixth nerve palsies. *Surv Ophthalmol.* 2009;54:305-310.

19. Takahashi H, Goto T, Shoji T, Tanito M, Park M, Chihara E. Diabetes-associated retinal nerve fiber damage evaluated with scanning laser polarimetry. *Am J Ophthalmol.* 2006;142:88-94.

20. Ganie MA, Bhat D. Current developments in Wolfram syndrome. *J Pediatr Endocrinol Metab.* 2009;22:3-10.

21. Lin CH, Lee YJ, Huang CY, et al. Wolfram (DIDMOAD) syndrome: report of two patients. *J Pediatr Endocrinol Metab.* 2004;17:1461-1464.

22. Tatham A. The relationship between diabetes mellitus and optic atrophy in children. *Diabet Med.* 2008;25:1486-1487.

23. Trigler L, Siatkowski RM, Oster AS, et al. Retinopathy in patients with diabetic ophthalmoplegia. *Ophthalmology.* 2003;110:1545-1550.

24. Kanazawa A, Haginomori S, Takamaki A, Nonaka R, Araki M, Takenaka H. Prognosis for Bell's palsy: a comparison of diabetic and nondiabetic patients. *Acta Otolaryngol.* 2007;127:888-891.

4

Diabetes Mellitus and the Cornea

Roberto Pineda, MD and Alejandro Espaillat, MD

The cornea is a transparent avascular tissue composed of 5 layers. It contains one of the highest concentrations of nerve endings in the body and is 100 times more sensitive than the conjunctiva.[1] This structure provides two-thirds of the refractive power of the eye, and dysfunction of this tissue can lead to loss of vision, pain, or both. Corneal nutrition is dependent on glucose from aqueous humor and oxygen from air; however, the peripheral cornea obtains glucose and oxygen from the limbal circulation. Thus, it is not surprising that diabetes mellitus affects all layers of the cornea, resulting in a number of pathologic conditions. Diabetic keratopathy has been reported to affect >50% of individuals.[2]

This chapter reviews the morphologic and physiologic implications of diabetes in the cornea, as well as its pathologic clinical manifestations. Newer technology, such as confocal microscopy and measurement of corneal hysteresis, has helped increase our understanding of the diabetic cornea.

CORNEAL EPITHELIUM AND DIABETES

The normal corneal epithelium is composed of 5 to 7 cell layers and is approximately 50 μm thick. A number of morphological changes in the diabetic corneal epithelium have been described, including fewer cells

and cell layers, thinning of the epithelium, and irregular surface cell microvilli.[3]

In the epithelial basement membrane, common morphological changes are thickening of the basement membrane, the presence of multiple layers, and areas of discontinuity.[4] Increased glycosylation of basement membrane components has been recognized for some time. A recent study by Kaji et al[5] evaluated advanced glycation end products (AGEs) in the diabetic cornea and their role in diabetic keratopathy. They used a monoclonal antibody to identify N-carboxymethyl lysine (CML) protein adducts. CML immunoreactivity was noted in the epithelial basement membrane of 8 diabetic corneas and only 1 of the controls (n = 8). Additionally, in vitro studies of nonenzymatic glycation of laminin attenuated spreading and adhesion of corneal epithelial cells in the culture dish. When aminoguanidine was added to the incubation mixture during glycation, CML formation was inhibited. This promoted the spreading and adhesion of culture dish corneal epithelial cells in a dose-dependent manner. This study reinforces the impact of AGEs, particularly laminin, a major component of the epithelial basement membrane, as an underlying pathologic cause of diabetic corneal epithelial disorders.[5] Aldose reductase is present in the corneal epithelium and has been associated with a number of ocular diabetic disorders.[6] It is the first enzyme of the polyol pathway and is another factor contributing to corneal epithelial and basement membrane disorders. Diabetic animal model studies evaluating the corneal

Espaillat A.
Diabetic Eye Disease: A Comprehensive Review (pp. 21-26)
© 2012 SLACK Incorporated

Table 4-1. Clinical Findings in Primary Diabetic Keratopathy		
Epithelium	• Superficial punctate keratopathy • Recurrent epithelial erosions • Chronic epitheliitis • Filamentary keratitis • Epithelial fragility	• Delayed epithelial healing • Persistent epithelial defects • Sterile ulcers • Microcystic edema and bleb formation
Descemet's Membrane	• Wrinkles (Waite-Beetham lines)	
Endothelium	• Unpigmented precipitates • Pigmentation	• Beaten-silver appearance

epithelial basement membrane have shown decreased membrane thickening and discontinuities using aldose reductase inhibitors.[7] Another study in diabetic rats showed faster epithelial healing after débridement compared to controls with the use of an aldose reductase inhibitor.[8]

Another clinical area that appears to be affected in the corneal epithelium of diabetics is corneal epithelial healing and adherence. Examination of the basement membrane complex in the diabetic cornea has identified abnormalities in multiple structures essential to proper adhesion of the basement membrane and epithelium to the stroma: hemidesmosomes, anchoring fibrils, and basal lamina.[9]

In the clinical setting, when the epithelium is removed in the diabetic cornea, the basement membrane often is removed with it. This can significantly delay healing as has been shown in studies with and without a normal basement membrane.[10] With the absence of a basement membrane, the synthesis and re-epithelialization can be substantially delayed (weeks). In the diabetic cornea, recovery is more likely prolonged.

Epithelial barrier function appears to be greatly altered in the diabetic cornea as well. This is relevant, as the epithelium's zonulae occludentes act as a diffusion barrier. Increased epithelial permeability appears to be common in diabetics and related to the duration of diabetes as well as the severity of diabetic retinopathy. One study noted that patients with proliferative and nonproliferative diabetic retinopathy were 84% and 41%, respectively, more likely to have corneal epithelial fragility than diabetics without retinopathy.[11]

With all of the epithelial and basement membrane changes, it is not surprising that Schultz et al[2] reported that 47% to 64% of diabetic patients suffer from primary diabetic corneal epitheliopathy during their lifetime. Table 4-1 lists the clinical manifestations of primary diabetic keratopathy.[12] Likewise, the diabetic corneal epithelium is highly susceptible to injury

during ocular surgery and in the postoperative period. In the late 1970s, corneal complications after pars plana vitrectomy largely occurred in diabetic patients and came to be known as postvitrectomy keratopathy. Fortunately, with improved surgical techniques, this rate has dropped significantly. Today, the most common manifestations of diabetic postvitrectomy keratopathy are delayed epithelialization and persistent epithelial defects.[13] Aldose reductase inhibitors have been used in human patients with variable success but are not currently in clinical use.

CORNEAL DIABETIC NEUROPATHY

As one of the principal tissues in the body with the highest concentration of nerve endings, it is no wonder that the cornea is so prominently affected by diabetes mellitus, and that diabetes damages corneal nerves.[14] Due to its avascular nature, the cornea may serve as a model for the nonvascular impact of diabetic neuropathy. Research has indicated that the nonmyelinated corneal nerves are first affected in diabetic neuropathy with irregularities in the nerve beading pattern and axonal degeneration of nonmyelinated corneal nerves, although abnormalities in the Schwann cell basal lamina have also been described.[15] Denervation of the diabetic cornea could affect the availability of cyclic adenosine monophosphate (cAMP) and cyclic guanosine monophosphate (cGMP), possibly affecting corneal epithelial mitosis and perhaps contributing to delayed epithelialization.

The use of confocal microscopy allows in vivo morphometric evaluation of the cornea and quantification of damage to corneal structures. Several studies have evaluated the sub-basal nerve plexus in diabetic patients using confocal microscopy. In a confocal microscopy study by Midena et al of the sub-basal nerve plexus, the number of fibers, number of beadings, and branching pattern of fibers were significantly decreased in diabetic eyes, whereas nerve tortuosity significantly increased.[16] A similar study correlated the degree of nerve tortuosity with the presence of proliferative diabetic retinopathy.[17]

It appears that corneal nerve morphologic changes on confocal microscopy also occur well ahead of corneal mechanical sensitivity. Previous studies have shown a decreased corneal sensation in the diabetic population, and it has been suggested that this can be used as a screening tool for diabetics. However, a confocal microscopy study by Rosenberg et al showed that loss of long nerve fiber bundles largely preceded impairment of corneal sensitivity, except in severe keratoneuropathy, and confocal microscopy may serve as a better predictor.[18]

The importance of corneal innervation for the maintenance of the corneal epithelium's function and structure is well documented. Decreased sensory input to the corneal epithelium leads to diminished cellular adhesion, impaired healing, and reduced mitosis. This is seen in other clinical conditions such as herpes simplex and herpes zoster keratitis, which greatly affect the corneal nerve plexus. In the diabetic cornea, additional changes in the corneal epithelium and basement membrane further compromise these corneas.

CORNEAL STROMA AND DIABETES

Although no major clinical disorders of the cornea are specifically ascribed to the stroma, the diabetic corneal stroma is abnormal. Experimental studies of the diabetic rat cornea show a decrease in the stromal collagen fibrils and increase in stromal proteoglycans. Furthermore, increased corneal cross-linking is present in the corneal stromal collagen. This biochemical cross-linking change has been demonstrated via the advanced Maillard reaction and occurs in the retina as well.

With such effects in the corneal stroma, biomechanical changes are expected. Two studies examined the diabetic cornea with the Ocular Response Analyzer (ORA; Reichert Technologies, Depew, NY) evaluating corneal hysteresis and corneal resistance factor as well as central corneal thickness.[19,20] Both studies found central corneal thickness to be increased. However, corneal hysteresis was lower in one study and higher in another, whereas corneal resistance factor was unchanged in one study and higher in the other. It is unclear at this point how diabetes affects corneal biomechanics. Further research is needed in this area.

DESCEMET'S MEMBRANE AND DIABETES

The classic hallmark of wrinkles in the Descemet's membrane in diabetic eyes has been described and referred to as "Waite-Beetham lines."[21] These lines were thought to be due to corneal hydration or associated with proliferative diabetic retinopathy. These lines have recently been described by confocal microscopy. Although the thickness of Descemet's membrane appears to be normal, histologic studies have identified more diabetic corneas with abnormal, posteriorly located banded material, similar to aphakic bullous keratopathy and Fuchs corneal dystrophy.

CORNEAL ENDOTHELIUM AND DIABETES

More recent studies of the endothelial cell density in diabetics have found a decrease in the endothelial cell count. This difference appears to be greater in patients with type 1 diabetes than type 2 diabetes. One study found an 11% reduction in type 1 diabetics, and a 5% reduction in type 2 diabetics compared to controls.[22] Endothelial morphometric changes also occur in both type 1 and type 2 diabetics (higher coefficient of variation, decreased percentage of hexagonal cells, increased polymegathism, decreased pleomorphism), and these changes are no different than age-related changes but tend to occur earlier, especially in type 1 diabetics. All of these morphologic corneal endothelial changes in the diabetic patient should signal that this cell layer is under continuous metabolic stress and is consequently highly vulnerable to insult.

The sorbitol pathway, and its osmotic effects, has been suggested as a mechanism to explain endothelial morphologic changes, as aldose reductase is found in the corneal endothelium. Additionally, hyperglycemia can inhibit endothelial sodium-potassium adenosine triphosphatase dependent transport (Na+/K+ ATPase)-dependent transport. This endothelial pump dysfunction has been described in an animal model with a 69% to 76% reduction of enzymatic activity leading to increased corneal hydration or loss of corneal deturgescence.[23] These findings could explain why in some studies the central corneal thickness is increased. Corneal permeability has been examined in several studies with mixed findings, showing it increased or with no difference when compared to controls.

DIABETES AND THE DRY EYE

Dry eye syndrome is a common problem among patients with diabetes. Several recent studies have documented its prevalence. It is generally believed that dry eye syndrome affects up to 50% of diabetic patients. Diabetic dry eye syndrome is largely due to aqueous tear deficiency as demonstrated in one study.[24] It is thought that dry eye syndrome in the diabetic patient is due to an autonomic neuropathy affecting the lacrimal gland, resulting in reduction of tear volume. However, as our understanding of the pathogenesis of dry eye expands, it is now known how disruption of the neural feedback loop affects the overall homeostasis of the ocular surface. Certainly, diabetic pathologic involvement of the corneal epithelium and sub-basal nerve plexus only further complicates the dry eye issue for these patients. The approach for treatment in the diabetic dry eye patient should be no different than for the typical dry eye patient. Medications such as 0.05% topical cyclosporine may be less effective due to the noninflammatory neuropathy occurring in these eyes.

CONTACT LENSES AND THE DIABETIC CORNEA

Because the cornea of diabetic patients is abnormal with an increased incidence of punctate keratitis and decreased corneal sensitivity, the question arises regarding the safety of contact lenses, as patients with diabetes have an increased risk of overall infection. Several studies have addressed this question and found no difference in contact lens complications between diabetic patients and controls using daily wear soft contact lenses. However, hard contact lenses as well as extended wear soft contact lenses are not recommended for diabetic patients due to the increased hypoxic stress on the cornea and mechanical trauma. Additionally, contact lenses are now being explored as a way to monitor blood glucose levels using nanoparticles embedded in hydrogel contact lenses that change hue when the blood glucose level is too high.

CORNEAL SURGERY IN THE DIABETIC PATIENT

By now, it is clear that the diabetic cornea is a vulnerable tissue that is easily stressed and susceptible to injury.

Avoidance of the corneal epithelium during surgery is critical while protection of the epithelium is equally paramount. The use of topical phenylephrine should be avoided in the presence of an epithelial defect as it can cause severe damage to the corneal endothelium. Any ocular procedure affecting the corneal epithelium or endothelium (pars plana vitrectomy, laser photocoagulation) may result in long-term complications to the cornea, necessitating additional corneal surgery.

In penetrating keratoplasty, it has been noted that when the donor's cornea is from a patient with diabetes, a significant risk exists for epithelial defects in the postoperative period.

Perhaps the ocular surgery most likely to impact the diabetic cornea is cataract surgery, as both the epithelium and endothelium can be adversely affected. In one early phacoemulsification study, corneal endothelial permeability in diabetic patients was no different preoperatively than controls, but endothelial diffusion barrier function took 6 weeks to recover in diabetic patients versus 3 weeks for controls. In 2 more recent studies regarding diabetic corneal endothelium after phacoemulsification, both showed greater loss of endothelial cell density. One study showed increased corneal thickness at 1 month in the diabetic patient, and the other demonstrated increased coefficient of variation for high-risk proliferative diabetic retinopathy.[25,26]

Currently, over 1 million refractive surgery procedures are performed in the United States every year. Laser in situ keratomileusis (LASIK), photorefractive keratectomy (PRK), and its related laser procedures are now commonplace. Diabetes may be considered a relative or absolute contraindication for laser vision correction depending on the status of the individual. Many studies about laser vision correction, and its safety and efficacy, are published in the literature; however, few have targeted the diabetic patient. One study in 2002 by Fraunfelder et al examined LASIK complications in patients with diabetes mellitus.[27] This study examined the 6-month microkeratome LASIK data of 30 eyes of patients with diabetes mellitus and 150 control eyes. They found that diabetic eyes had a 47% complication rate compared with a 7% control complication rate. The most frequent complications were punctate epithelial erosions and persistent epithelial defects. In addition, diabetic patients had poorer refractive outcomes than controls.

In another study of 24 well-controlled diabetic patients who had LASIK surgery from one center with median 6-month follow-up, 29 eyes (63%) achieved an uncorrected visual acuity of 20/25 or better, and 31 eyes (67%) were within ±0.50 diopters of the intended refraction after the first LASIK surgery.[28] Retreatment was required in 13 eyes (28%) because initial surgery was not adequate to correct the refractive error. Three eyes (7%) developed an epithelial defect after surgery, and secondary epithelial ingrowth developed in 2 of these eyes. It was concluded that LASIK was safe in well-controlled diabetics but that enhancements may be required more often.

SUMMARY

Diabetes mellitus affects all layers of the cornea. It has morphologic, metabolic, and physiologic consequences with significant clinical manifestations. It is important to understand the implications of this disease for both the treatment of corneal disorders and ocular-related surgery. The corneal epithelium and endothelium are particularly stressed in the diabetic cornea, even without insult. Corneal innervation is notably affected in diabetes, and the biomechanics of the cornea, particularly the stroma, appear to be altered. Changes in the diabetic cornea may correlate with the severity and duration of the disease. Patients with diabetic corneal disease should be approached cautiously to minimize further damage to an already delicate and fragile tissue.

REFERENCES

1. Muller LJ, Vrensen GFJM, Pels L, Cardozo BN, Willekens B. Architecture of human corneal nerves. *Invest Ophthalmol Vis Sci.* 1997;38:985-994.
2. Schultz RO, Peters MA, Sobocinski K, et al. Diabetic corneal neuropathy. *Trans Am Ophthalmol Soc.* 1983;81:107-124.
3. Tsubota K, Chiba K, Shimazaki J. Corneal epithelium in diabetic patients. *Cornea.* 1991;10:156-160.
4. Taylor HR, Kimsey RA. Corneal epithelial basement membrane changes in diabetes. *Invest Ophthalmol Vis Sci.* 1981;20:548-553.
5. Kaji Y, Usui T, Oshika T, et al. Advanced glycation end products in diabetic corneas. *Invest Ophthalmol Vis Sci.* 2000;41:362-368.
6. Kern TS, Engerman RL. Distribution of aldose reductase in ocular tissues. *Exp Eye Res.* 1981;33:175-182.
7. Kodama Y, Akagi Y, Sasamoto K, et al. Effects of an aldose reductase inhibitor on ocular tissues of diabetic rats. *Folia Ophthalmol Jpn.* 1984;35:740-748.
8. Fukushi S, Merola LO, Tanaka M. Reepithelialization of denuded corneas in diabetic rats. *Exp Eye Res.* 1980;31:611-621.
9. Gipson IK, Spurr-Mirchaud SJ, Tisdale AS. Anchoring fibrils form a complex network in human and rabbit cornea. *Invest Ophthalmol Vis Sci.* 1987;289:212-221.
10. Khodadoust AA, Silverstein AM, Kenyon K, et al. Adhesion of regenerating corneal epithelium. The role of basement membrane. *Am J Ophthalmol.* 1968;65:339-348.
11. Saini JS, Khandalavia B. Corneal epithelial fragility in diabetes mellitus. *Can J Ophthalmol.* 1995;30:142-146.
12. Sanchez-Thorin JC. The cornea in diabetes mellitus. *Int Ophthalmol Clin.* 1998;38:19-36.
13. Perry HD, Foulks GN, Thoft RA, Tolentino FI. Corneal complications following closed vitrectomy through the pars plana. *Arch Ophthalmol.* 1978;96:1401-1403.
14. Schultz RO, Peters MA, Sobocinski K, et al. Diabetic keratopathy as a manifestation of peripheral neuropathy. *Am J Ophthalmol.* 1983;96:368-371.
15. Ishida N, Rao GN, Del Cerro M, Aquavella JV. Corneal nerve alterations in diabetes mellitus. *Arch Ophthalmol.* 1984;102:1380-1384.
16. Midena E, Cortese M, Miotto S, Gambato C, Cavarzeran F, Ghirlando A. Confocal microscopy of corneal sub-basal nerve plexus: a quantitative and qualitative analysis in healthy and pathologic eyes. *J Refract Surg.* 2009;25(1 Suppl):S125-130.
17. Midena E, Brugin E, Ghirlando A, Sommavilla M, Avogaro A. Corneal diabetic neuropathy: a confocal microscopy study. *J Refract Surg.* 2006;22(9 Supp):S1047-1052.
18. Rosenberg ME, Tervo TM, Müller LJ, Moilanen JA, Vesaluoma MH. In vivo confocal microscopy after herpes keratitis. *Cornea.* 2002;21(3):265-269.
19. Kotecha A, Oddone F, Sinapis C, et al. Corneal biomechanical characteristics in patients with diabetes mellitus. *J Cataract Refract Surg.* 2010;36(11):1822-1828.
20. Goldich Y, Barkana Y, Gerber Y, et al. Effect of diabetes mellitus on biomechanical parameters of the cornea. *J Cataract Refract Surg.* 2009;35(4):715-719.
21. Mocan MC, Irkeç M, Orhan M. Evidence of Waite-Beetham lines in the cornea of diabetic patients as detected by in vivo confocal microscopy. *Eye.* 2006;20(12):1488-1490. Epub 2006 Apr 28.
22. Larson LI, Bourne WM, Pach JM, Brubaker RF. Structure and function of the corneal endothelium in diabetes mellitus type I and type II. *Arch Ophthalmol.* 1996;114(1):9-14.
23. Shenoy R, Khandekar R, Bialasiewicz A, Al Muniri A. Corneal endothelium in patients with diabetes mellitus: a historical cohort study. *Eur J Ophthalmol.* 2009;19(3):369-375.
24. Akinci A, Cetinkaya E, Aycan Z. Dry eye syndrome in diabetic children. *Eur J Ophthalmol.* 2007;17(6):873-878.
25. Hugod M, Storr-Paulsen A, Norregaard JC, Nicolini J, Larsen AB, Thulesen J. Corneal endothelial cell changes associated with cataract surgery in patients with type 2 diabetes mellitus. *Cornea.* 2011;30(7):749-753.
26. Lee JS, Lee JE, Choi HY, Oum BS, Cho BM. Corneal endothelial cell change after phacoemulsification relative to the severity of diabetic retinopathy. *J Cataract Refractive Surg.* 2005;31(4):742-749.
27. Fraunfelder FW, Rich LF. Laser-assisted in situ keratomileusis complications in diabetes mellitus. *Cornea.* 2002;21(3):246-248.
28. Halkiadakis I, Belfair N, Gimbel HV. Laser in situ keratomileusis in patients with diabetes. *J Cataract Refract Surg.* 2005;31(10):1895-1898.

5

Diabetes Mellitus and Cataracts

Cecilia R. Sanchez, MD; Sabera T. Shah, MD; Timothy J. Murtha, MD; and Alejandro Espaillat, MD

EPIDEMIOLOGY

Diabetes affected approximately 285 million people worldwide and over 24 million people in the United States alone in 2010. It is expected to affect 439 million people worldwide by the year 2030 (Table 5-1).[1] Given this epidemic of diabetes, diabetic eye complications can be expected to rise. Currently, the overall 25-year incidence of visual impairment (visual acuity of 20/40 or worse) is 13%, and the incidence of severe visual impairment (20/200 or worse) is 3% among patients with type 1 diabetes in the United States.[2] According to a recent Wisconsin Epidemiologic Study of Diabetic Retinopathy (WESDR) report, cataracts, more severe baseline diabetic retinopathy, higher HbA1C, hypertension, and smoking are strongly associated with a risk for visual impairment among patients with diabetes.[2] Individuals with diabetes are 2 to 5 times more likely to develop cataracts than those without diabetes and do so at an earlier age.[3-6]

The Early Treatment Diabetic Retinopathy Study (ETDRS) and WESDR study on the incidence of cataract surgery in patients with diabetes report an increased risk for cataracts and/or cataract surgery associated with increased age, female gender, smoking, and proteinuria.[3,7] According to the WESDR study, patients with type 1 diabetes and advanced diabetic retinopathy at the time of enrollment in the study had a greater risk for subsequent cataract surgery. Older onset patients with diabetes who used insulin were also at higher risk for cataracts.[3] In the ETDRS, a history of vitrectomy increased the risk of cataract surgery 7-fold.[7] It has been suggested by several authors that early or accelerated development of cataracts may be an indicator of more advanced diabetes.[7-9]

PATHOPHYSIOLOGY OF DIABETIC CATARACTS

With hyperglycemia, excess glucose from the aqueous diffuses into the lens where some of it is converted to sorbitol through the aldose reductase pathway. The excess sorbitol is not readily converted to fructose and accumulates in the lens, causing an increase in the osmotic pressure gradient with an influx of fluid into the lens and resultant swelling of the crystalline lens. This disruption of the normal protein structure of the lens causes cortical vacuoles and opacification.[10,11] As blood and aqueous glucose levels rise and fall, rapid changes in the hydration of the lens may also cause transient myopia or hyperopia associated with uncontrolled diabetes or institution of intensive glycemic control.[12,13]

Espaillat A.
Diabetic Eye Disease: A Comprehensive Review (pp. 27-40)
© 2012 SLACK Incorporated

Table 5-1. Global Projections for the Diabetes Epidemic: 2010-2030			
	2010 (millions)	*2030 (millions)*	*2010-2030 % Increase*
North America and Caribbean	37.4	53.2	42
Central America and South America	18.0	29.6	65
Europe	55.2	66.2	20
Africa	12.1	23.9	98
Middle East and North Africa	26.2	51.7	97
South-East Asia	58.7	101.0	72
Western Pacific	76.7	112.8	47
World	284.3	438.4	54

Following vitrectomy surgery, posterior subcapsular cataracts and nuclear sclerotic cataracts develop in approximately 75% of patients with diabetes.[14,15] Posterior subcapsular cataract may result from trauma to the lens during vitrectomy. Development of nuclear sclerotic cataracts following vitrectomy surgery may be due to increased oxygen levels in the vitreous cavity following vitrectomy.[16] Interestingly, the incidence of postvitrectomy nuclear cataracts among patients with diabetes is lower than in postvitrectomy patients without diabetes.[17] Some authors speculate that lower oxygen tension in diabetic eyes may actually protect the lens from developing nuclear sclerotic cataracts in both vitrectomized and unoperated eyes.[18]

TYPES OF DIABETIC CATARACTS

Patients with diabetes may present with a variety of lens opacities (Figure 5-1). Although unusual in the United States today, the true diabetic cataract or snowflake cataract has subcapsular opacities in the anterior and posterior cortex and usually presents and progresses rapidly. This cataract typically occurs in young patients, as young as age 5, with uncontrolled or undiagnosed diabetes.[19-22] These acute onset cataracts may be reversible with glycemic control.[23,24] Another type of cataract associated with type 1 diabetes is the "Christmas tree" cataract, which may not impact vision and may not be an indication for surgery. Other typical lens opacities in patients with diabetes include cortical clefts and vacuoles[25] and posterior subcapsular cataracts.[26,27] Patients may also develop a nuclear sclerotic cataract,[5] although some studies have shown that patients with diabetes may actually have a lower risk of

nuclear sclerotic cataract compared to patients without diabetes.[25]

CATARACT SURGERY

Indications

Indications for cataract surgery in patients with diabetes can be complex. The visual needs of the patient must be balanced against the status of retinopathy. Patient symptoms may include standard cataract symptoms such as blurred vision, glare, haze, halo, reduced contrast sensitivity, and reduced color vision. However, some of these symptoms may result from or may be exacerbated by active retinopathy or prior laser photocoagulation treatment. As a result of symptoms induced by retinopathy or prior treatments, it often is appropriate to consider cataract intervention sooner than otherwise might be indicated with the hope of maximizing visual potential in an already compromised eye. Appropriate timing for cataract surgery could help maintain patient independence, ability to work, quality of life, and safety.

Management of diabetic retinopathy may impact the timing of cataract surgery. In some instances, lens opacity, whether symptomatic or not, may preclude adequate visualization of the retina. In these situations, cataract surgery may be necessary for diagnostic as well as therapeutic purposes.[28,29] On the other hand, symptomatic patients with active retinopathy or macular edema may require deferral of cataract surgery until appropriate treatment for retinopathy can be administered. Only after the macular edema is resolved or proliferative retinopathy becomes quiescent would it be reasonable to proceed with cataract surgery.

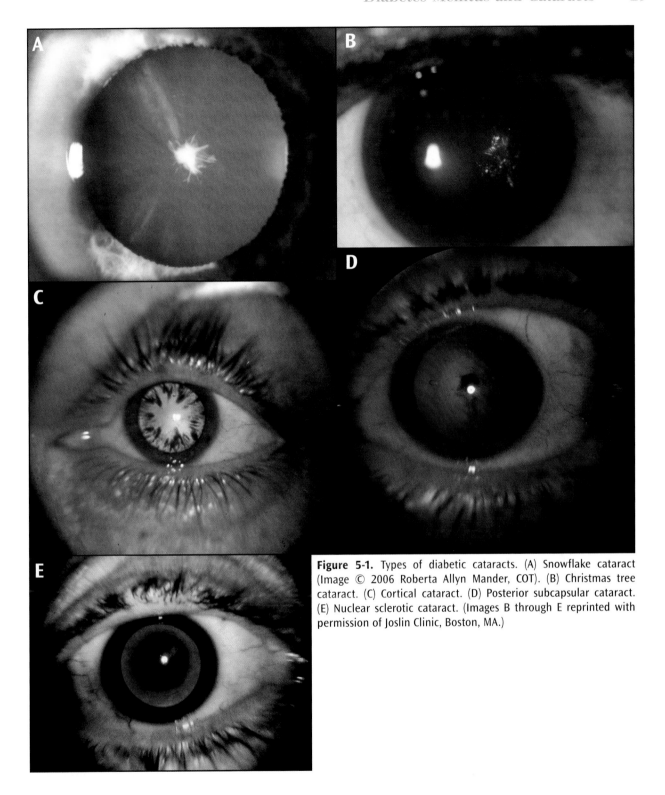

Figure 5-1. Types of diabetic cataracts. (A) Snowflake cataract (Image © 2006 Roberta Allyn Mander, COT). (B) Christmas tree cataract. (C) Cortical cataract. (D) Posterior subcapsular cataract. (E) Nuclear sclerotic cataract. (Images B through E reprinted with permission of Joslin Clinic, Boston, MA.)

In patients with diabetes, the cause of vision loss often is multifactorial and may be due to cataracts as well as macular or retinal pathology. Use of potential acuity meter (PAM) testing may be helpful for estimating postoperative visual outcome.[30] The results of PAM testing can be used to guide the surgical decision and counsel patients regarding a reasonable expected visual outcome.

As recently as the late 1980s and early 1990s, some surgeons deferred cataract surgery in patients with diabetic retinopathy until the vision was 20/100 to 20/200 or worse.[31] This delay was attributable to a number of studies demonstrating that postoperative visual acuity results were much worse in patients with diabetes, particularly those with any retinopathy.[32-34] One study in 1994 reported as few as 9% of patients with diabetes achieving visual acuity of 20/40 or better after sur-gery.[35] Fortunately, with newer surgical techniques and equipment, better medical management of diabetes, and improved management of diabetic retinopathy, patients are enjoying superior visual outcomes.

Visual Outcome

In general, patients with diabetes undergoing cataract surgery will appreciate some improvement in vision. In addition, although difficult to measure, many patients appreciate an enhancement of visual function, including improvement in glare, contrast, night vision, and color vision. After phacoemulsification, up to 85% of patients with diabetes will improve 2 lines[36-38] of visual acuity and up to 96% will have 1-year postoperative vision of 20/40 or better.[36-40] Some studies suggest worse visual outcome associated with poor preoperative visual acuity,[7] older age,[34] poor glycemic control (worsening retinopathy leading to worse visual outcome),[41] and extracapsular cataract extraction (ECCE) as compared to phacoemulsification.[40]

The best predictor of visual outcome after cataract surgery is preoperative level of retinopathy. Multiple studies have reported worse visual outcomes in eyes with more advanced diabetic retinopathy.[7,30,37,40,42,43] Somaiya and coworkers[30] reported that eyes with any level of nonproliferative diabetic retinopathy (NPDR) were nearly 5 times less likely and eyes with prolifera-tive diabetic retinopathy (PDR) were 30 times less likely to achieve postoperative visual acuity of 20/40 or better compared to patients without retinopathy. Eyes with active PDR have worse visual outcomes than those with quiescent PDR[44] and are also at higher risk for postop-erative complications such as vitreous hemorrhage or retinal detachment. Eyes with diabetic retinopathy are more likely to have macular edema pre- and postopera-tively. The presence of preoperative macular edema may be associated with worse visual outcome, even if focal macular laser was applied preoperatively.[34,45]

A retrospective subanalysis of original ETDRS data described visual outcome in patients with diabetes who underwent intracapsular cataract extraction (ICCE), ECCE, or phacoemulsification. ETDRS reported an improvement of 2 or more lines in 49% of operated eyes assigned to deferred photocoagulation and 64% of operated eyes that underwent early laser. One year post-operative best corrected visual acuity (BCVA) of 20/40 or better was achieved by 36% of eyes that underwent deferred laser and 46% in the early laser group.[7] Timing of laser was not a significant risk factor, although early scatter laser was associated with less severe retinopathy before surgery. The ETDRS found that more severe diabetic retinopathy and decreased preoperative visual acuity were significant risk factors for poor visual results after cataract surgery. One-year postoperative

visual acuity of better than 20/40 was achieved by 53% of eyes with baseline mild to moderate NPDR compared to 25% of eyes that had severe or worse NPDR or PDR. The inclusion of patients who underwent older tech-niques of cataract surgery (ICCE) probably contributed to lower rates of visual improvement compared to rates reported in more recent literature.

Some studies have shown better visual acuity out-comes after phacoemulsification compared to ECCE. Dowler et al compared phacoemulsification and ECCE in diabetic patients and reported visual acuity 20/40 or better in 96% of those who underwent phacoemul-sification compared to 83% of those who underwent ECCE.[40] Despite the shift toward smaller incisions, shorter duration surgeries, and the relatively good visual acuity outcomes achieved by patients with diabetes, the outcomes may not be comparable to patients without diabetes. Somaiya and coauthors reported postoperative visual acuity 20/40 or better after phacoemulsification in 82% of patients with diabetes compared to 95% without diabetes.[30]

Preoperative Considerations

Preoperative evaluation is an essential step for optimizing successful outcomes of cataract surgery in patients with diabetes. In addition to obtaining a detailed medical and ophthalmic history, the patient's history of diabetic retinopathy, neovascularization of the iris, macular edema, and previous laser or vitreoret-inal surgery should be considered, as these conditions may affect the potential outcome and expectations.

Preoperative medical evaluation is a controversial area in current cataract surgery practice. Several stud-ies have suggested that preoperative medical evalua-tion does not improve safety and may not be neces-sary for patients undergoing cataract surgery.[46-48] Although medical history may have less significance for patients without diabetes, experience at the Beetham Eye Institute of the Joslin Diabetes Center suggests that preoperative medical evaluation contributes to the suc-cess of the total management of patients with diabetes. Preoperative evaluation may provide motivation for patients to optimize glycemic control and also allows for the evaluation of diabetic comorbidities. Preoperative electrocardiogram may detect silent ischemic events that may not have been discovered otherwise and may precipitate further evaluation. Proactive medical man-agement in the setting of diabetes can prevent serious medical complications in the perioperative period and maximize the visual benefits.

Preoperative evaluation and treatment of macular edema and retinopathy are mandatory for planning the timing of cataract surgery. There are few recent studies investigating the timing of scatter laser photocoagula-tion in patients who will undergo cataract surgery. The

Table 5-2. Management of Diabetic Retinopathy Prior to Cataract Surgery

A.

Mild NPDR

Observe; proceed with cataract surgery

*ETDRS standard photograph 2A

B.

Moderate NPDR

Observe; proceed with cataract surgery

*ETDRS standard photograph 2B

C.

Severe or Very Severe NPDR

Early panretinal photocoagulation (PRP; especially if type 2 diabetes mellitus); stabilize for 3 to 6 months before cataract surgery

*ETDRS standard photograph 6B

D.

PDR, HRC or non-HRC

PRP; stabilize for 3 to 6 months before cataract surgery

*ETDRS standard photograph 10C

E.

Quiescent PDR

Observe; proceed with cataract surgery

*Photograph montage of patient with prior PRP

(Images A through D are reprinted with permission of Fundus Photograph Reading Center, University of Wisconsin—Madison, http://eyephoto.ophth.wisc.edu/ResearchAreas/Diabetes/DiabStds.htm. Image E is reprinted with permission of Joslin Clinic, Boston, MA.)

ETDRS reported better visual outcomes than other studies at the time, which may be in part due to earlier scatter laser photocoagulation. The ETDRS recommended scatter laser photocoagulation before cataract surgery for patients with PDR and severe NPDR.[7] In patients with active PDR, vitreous hemorrhage, or active neovascularization of the iris (NVI), intravitreal anti-VEGF agents can be considered prior to surgery (Table 5-2).

Figure 5-2. OCT images of cataract surgery with intravitreal steroid injection for refractory CSME. (A) Preoperative/pre-injection. (B) Three months status post-cataract surgery and intravitreal triamcinolone. (Images reprinted with permission of Joslin Clinic, Boston, MA.)

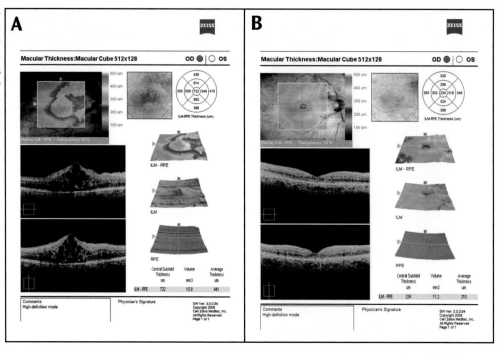

The presence of macular edema at the time of surgery is associated with worse visual outcomes[34]; therefore, evaluation of macular edema and consideration of treatment prior to surgery is crucial. Current standard of care suggests waiting 3 to 6 months after laser treatment for resolution of macular edema involving or threatening the center of the macula before proceeding with cataract surgery. A recent Diabetic Retinopathy Clinical Research Network (DRCR.net) study reported that intravitreal ranibizumab with prompt or deferred laser is more effective than laser alone for center-involved macular edema.[49] In cases where the cataract precludes focal laser, or the diabetic macular edema is persistent, intravitreal injection of anti-VEGF agents or steroids can be considered prior to, during, or after surgery. Recent studies suggest that intravitreal bevacizumab at the time of cataract surgery may promote better visual outcome and prevent progression of retinopathy.[50,51] Several small scale studies on intravitreal triamcinolone at the time of cataract surgery in patients with pre-existing clinically significant macular edema (CSME) demonstrated some improvement in macular thickness within the first few months postoperatively.[52,53] Lam and coauthors found that the effect was transient.[52] This was consistent with the findings of recent DRCR.net studies showing a rapid but short-term benefit of intravitreal triamcinolone compared with focal/grid laser for diabetic macular edema (Figure 5-2).[54] Larger scale, controlled studies with longer follow-up are necessary to determine which interventions will increase visual outcomes in patients with diabetes undergoing cataract surgery (Table 5-3).

Preoperative optical coherence tomography (OCT) and fluorescein angiography can be valuable in planning cataract surgery. In the setting of media opacity, OCT may identify visually significant epiretinal membrane or vitreomacular traction that may not be appreciated on clinical examination. The surgeon and patient may then consider scheduling a pars plana vitrectomy and membrane peeling at the time or after cataract surgery. Subtle macular edema may be identified on preoperative OCT, and as a result, the surgeon may consider additional treatment for macular edema pre- or intraoperatively. Similarly, fluorescein angiography may identify macular nonperfusion, which might limit postoperative visual potential (Figure 5-3).

In addition to preoperative medical and glycemic control and treatment of diabetic macular edema or retinopathy, preventative measures to reduce postoperative inflammation and infection may improve surgical outcomes.[8] Some surgeons advocate the use of topical non-steroidal anti-inflammatory drugs (NSAIDs) for 3 to 7 days preoperatively to reduce inflammation and risk of macular edema, especially in patients with diabetes who are at increased risk of postoperative inflammation and already have a compromised blood aqueous barrier.[8] NSAIDs may be beneficial in the setting of current or prior macular edema in the operative eye or history of postoperative macular edema in the fellow eye. Additionally, topical NSAIDs prolong the mydriatic effect of the dilating drops used perioperatively.[55] Some surgeons also use topical fourth-generation fluoroquinolones preoperatively for 1 to 7 days to minimize the bacterial load on the ocular surface and reduce the risk of endophthalmitis.[8]

Table 5-3. Management of Diabetic Macular Edema Prior to Cataract Surgery

A.	**Clinically significant macular edema (CSME)** Focal laser and/or intravitreal anti-VEGF agent prior to surgery; stabilize 3 to 6 months before cataract surgery *Photograph of hard exudates and CSME
B.	**Persistent CSME without vitreoretinal interface abnormality** Repeat treatment; stabilize 3 to 6 months before cataract surgery *OCT of CSME with cystoid spaces
C.	**Resolved or persistent diabetic macular edema (DME)** Pre-treat with topical NSAIDs *Fluorescein angiogram of prior laser treatment and persistent leakage
D.	**Persistent DME obscured by cataract** Adjunctive perioperative therapy: a. Vitrectomy b. Intravitreal anti-VEGF agent c. Intravitreal steroids d. Topical NSAIDS *Photograph of CSME and hard exudates with view limited by media opacity

(Images reprinted with permission of Joslin Clinic, Boston, MA.)

Operative Considerations

Phacoemulsification has become the preferred method for cataract surgery by most surgeons. Improved instrumentation and better phacoemulsification technique have reduced surgical trauma, duration, and light exposure, which is beneficial for surgical outcomes in patients with diabetes.[37,40] Dowler et al[40] compared phacoemulsification and ECCE in patients with diabetes. Patients who underwent ECCE had more inflammation 1 week postoperatively and were more likely to have intraocular lens (IOL) deposits and need YAG capsulotomy. Both methods of cataract surgery produced excellent visual outcomes. However, vision was slightly better after phacoemulsification than ECCE (20/20 versus 20/25). No difference was observed in incidence of postoperative CSME or progression of retinopathy after phacoemulsification compared to ECCE.[40]

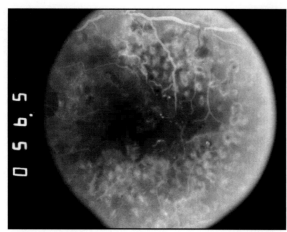

Figure 5-3. Fluorescein angiogram with prior laser treatment and macular nonperfusion. (Reprinted with permission of Joslin Clinic, Boston, MA.)

INTRAOCULAR LENS SELECTION

In choosing an IOL for a patient with diabetes, the material, style, and refractive goal should be considered. The most commonly used lenses are made from silicone, polymethylmethacrylate (PMMA), and acrylic. Silicone lenses should be avoided in patients with silicone oil in the posterior chamber or those likely to need it in the future because oil adheres to silicone IOLs. There is also increased condensation on silicone IOLs during vitrectomy with fluid-air exchange. Furthermore, some studies suggest that silicone IOLs may stimulate inflammation in diabetic eyes; therefore, acrylic IOLs or heparin-coated PMMA IOLs may be preferred.[56,57] In addition, appropriate adjustment of IOL calculations must be made for eyes containing silicone oil.

Careful consideration of the use of multifocal and accommodating IOLs in patients with diabetes is important. These lenses can create challenges for a retinal surgeon during any subsequent retinal surgery. The Crystalens (Eyeonics, Aliso Viejo, CA) is an accommodating, monofocal, silicone IOL that should be avoided in eyes that may later require silicone oil. Additionally, if a patient requires vitrectomy with air-fluid exchange, the surgery can cause movement of the lens, pushing it forward, affecting the function of the Crystalens, which requires proper positioning within the capsular bag. Multifocal IOLs can impair the retinal surgeon's visualization and stereopsis during vitreoretinal surgery.[58]

Some presbyopia-correcting IOLs may also limit the postoperative vision of patients with diabetes. Multifocal IOLs may allow excellent uncorrected visual acuity in patients with no underlying ocular pathology[59] as well as patients with diabetic retinopathy.[60] However, they may decrease contrast sensitivity in patients with no concurrent eye disease.[61,62] This decrease is probably clinically insignificant for most patients,[63] but for those with diabetes who may already have compromised contrast sensitivity resulting from laser treatment, retinopathy, nonperfusion,[64] or reduced visual potential, careful consideration is warranted. Use of a blue-light filtering IOL in patients with diabetes may provide better contrast sensitivity than standard acrylic IOLs,[65] so use of these lenses may be acceptable. Aspheric IOLs may also provide better contrast sensitivity,[66,67] although this use has not been tested specifically in patients with diabetes.

In patients with diabetes with compromised vision and limited visual potential resulting from diabetic eye disease, it may be preferable to calculate IOL powers that would result in a mild to moderate myopic result to facilitate and complement low vision correction postoperatively.

COMBINED VITRECTOMY AND CATARACT SURGERY

Standard phacoemulsification surgery in patients with advanced diabetic eye disease can be complemented with the addition of vitrectomy surgery to maximize visual potential. The most common indications for pars plana vitrectomy in patients with diabetes include nonclearing vitreous hemorrhage, traction retinal detachment, vitreomacular traction, epiretinal membrane, and refractory CSME (Figure 5-4). If lens opacity impairs the retinal surgeon's view or is likely to progress significantly after vitreoretinal surgery, cataract extraction with IOL placement can be combined with pars plana vitrectomy. Studies have shown that this combined procedure can be performed safely and effectively in patients with diabetes.[68-70] Advantages of a combined procedure include better visualization of the posterior pole during vitrectomy and a single operation, which may reduce patient discomfort, costs, and recovery time.[71] Combined cataract-vitrectomy surgery eliminates some difficulties of performing cataract surgery on a previously vitrectomized eye, including a soft eye, deep anterior chamber, excessively mobile posterior capsule, and decreased zonular support, which increase the risk of posterior capsule rupture.[72,73] Caution should be used in undertaking combined cataract-vitrectomy surgery in certain situations. In settings where the red reflex is compromised, difficulties in visualizing the capsulorrhexis and subsequent placement of the IOL may be experienced. Additionally, anterior segment manipulation may result in pupillary miosis, bleeding, decreased corneal clarity, IOL decentration, and retained air bubbles, which may impair ideal visualization for subsequent vitrectomy surgery.[71,74,75]

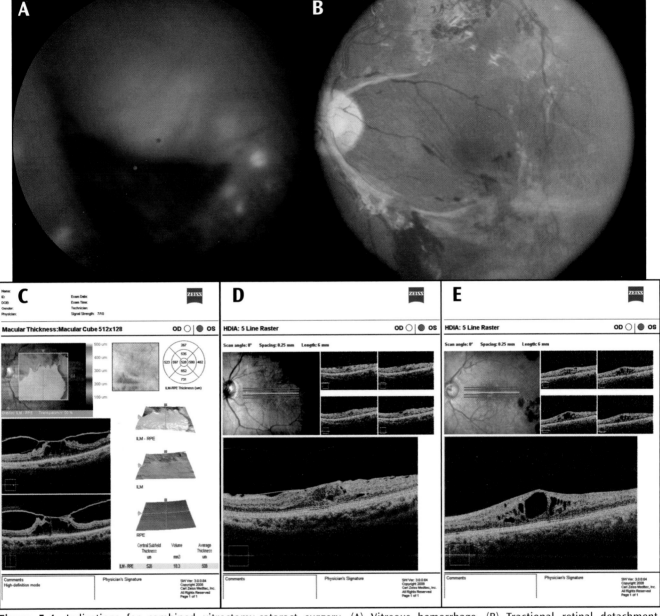

Figure 5-4. Indications for combined vitrectomy-cataract surgery. (A) Vitreous hemorrhage. (B) Tractional retinal detachment. (C) Vitreomacular traction. (D) Epiretinal membrane. (E) Persistent/refractory macular edema. (Images reprinted with permission of Joslin Clinic, Boston, MA.)

Intraoperative Considerations

In addition to difficulties of operating on a previously vitrectomized eye, other intraoperative challenges are faced by the cataract surgeon operating on a patient with diabetes. These patients may dilate poorly due to ischemia, neuropathy of sympathetic innervation, or changes in the dilator muscle.[76-79] Preoperative topical NSAIDs may prolong the mydriatic effect of dilating drops. Intraoperatively, the surgeon can use high molecular weight viscoelastic solutions, gentle pupil stretching, and iris hooks or pupillary expansion rings to enlarge the pupil and improve visualization.

The pupil may not dilate well if the pupillary margin has synechiae or is fibrotic due to active or regressed NVI. In these cases, it is important to avoid excessive manipulation of the iris, as bleeding during the surgery or postoperatively is a risk, as well as increased inflammation. Patients with diabetes frequently suffer from corneal epithelial injuries resulting in corneal erosions, edema, haze, or epithelial breakdown, causing difficulty in visualization during the procedure.

With appropriate preoperative evaluation, treatment, and planning, and with careful, deliberate actions during cataract surgery, some intraoperative complications can be avoided or minimized.

Postoperative Complications

Patients with diabetes are more likely to have more intense postoperative inflammation and may even develop sterile endophthalmitis. Inflammation often is more severe after longer surgeries, and in extreme cases, membranous uveitis may develop after ECCE in patients with diabetes. Inflammation may be more severe in complicated cases with posterior capsule rupture and vitreous loss.

Studies suggest that patients with diabetes have a higher risk of developing postoperative endophthalmitis compared to those without diabetes. Previous studies have reported that 14% to 21% of patients with endophthalmitis had diabetes,[80,81] which may be due to impaired immune response or delayed wound healing. Patients with diabetes present similarly to those without diabetes, with pain reported by 78% to 85%. They may be more likely to develop a hypopyon compared to patients without diabetes. Patients with diabetes are more likely to have positive cultures and a slight tendency to culture more virulent organisms than patients without diabetes.[80-82] Visual outcome after endophthalmitis is also worse in patients with diabetes, particularly those with pre-existing retinopathy.[80] Phillips and coauthors reported no light perception vision in up to 30% of patients with diabetes treated for postoperative endophthalmitis.[81] The Endophthalmitis Vitrectomy Study reported that 39% of patients with diabetes treated for postoperative endophthalmitis achieved a final visual acuity of 20/40 compared to 55% of nondiabetic patients. Regardless of diabetes status, patients with initial vision of light perception had a better visual outcome with immediate vitrectomy. When initial vision was better than light perception, patients with diabetes achieved vision of 20/40 or better often after vitrectomy (57%) than after tap/inject (40%), although this difference was not statistically significant. In contrast, patients without diabetes did equally well with vitrectomy or tap/inject.[82] Therefore, more aggressive intervention in patients with diabetes and endophthalmitis may be appropriate.

Patients with diabetes are at higher risk for postoperative complications. The incidence of posterior capsular opacity is slightly higher in these patients compared to patients without diabetes[83] regardless of the level of retinopathy or systemic control.[84] Patients with diabetes, in particular those with retinopathy, also have a tendency for anterior capsule contraction.[85,86] YAG capsulotomy may be indicated in the early postoperative period. However, if active macular edema or retinopathy is present, deferral of the capsulotomy should be considered until retinopathy is stabilized with laser therapy or pharmaceuticals.

The presence of NVI may result in postoperative hyphema with associated intraocular pressure elevation.

Intraocular pressure needs to be managed with aggressive topical therapy, and the patient will need scatter laser photocoagulation as soon as possible. Alternatively, many physicians have begun to use intravitreal bevacizumab, often in combination with scatter laser photocoagulation, to treat neovascularization of the iris or angle,[87-89] and this appears to be well tolerated in the postoperative period. Postoperative intraocular pressure spikes are not unusual. However, in patients with diabetes who have compromised retinal vascular flow and nonperfusion, more aggressive and early control of intraocular pressure may be warranted.

Although current trends for postoperative follow-up are moving toward fewer postoperative visits, a closer follow-up after cataract surgery may be indicated in patients with diabetes given the higher risk for the development of serious complications.

MANAGEMENT OF POSTOPERATIVE DIABETIC MACULAR EDEMA

Macular edema as a consequence of cataract surgery in patients with diabetes is controversial. Pollack et al reported angiographic cystoid macular edema (CME) in 50% of patients with diabetes compared to 8% without diabetes after ECCE.[31] Review of the literature suggests that the incidence of postoperative macular edema in patients with diabetes is in the range of 7% to >50%.[31,36,39,40,90] The ETDRS found no significant difference in rate of macular edema after surgery[7] and other studies found no difference in macular edema in operated eyes compared to nonoperated eyes.[38,90] On the other hand, several other studies have noted higher rates of postoperative macular edema among those with pre-existing retinopathy.[31,36,39,91]

The wide range of reported incidence of macular edema may be due to unrecognized preoperative edema. Also, it can be difficult to differentiate postoperative pseudophakic CME (Irvine-Gass) from diabetic macular edema, and there may be components of both. Fluorescein angiography demonstrating a hyperfluorescent macula in a petaloid pattern and absence of retinopathy or microaneurysms is suggestive of Irvine-Gass edema. Hyperfluorescence of the disc may also characterize Irvine-Gass edema, although some authors believe that this is not predictive or specific.[39] Hard exudates or microaneurysms and hemorrhages in the macula are more suggestive of diabetic macular edema (Figure 5-5). Irvine-Gass macular edema tends to resolve[92] whereas diabetic macular edema, especially if present preoperatively, has a tendency to progress.[93] In

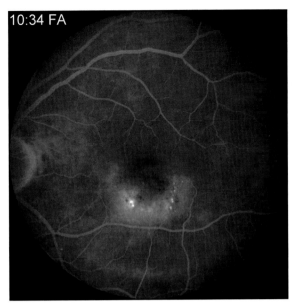

Figure 5-5. Fluorescein angiogram of CSME. (Reprinted with permission of Joslin Clinic, Boston, MA.)

Several studies have found no significant difference in the rate of retinopathy progression after phacoemulsification compared to ECCE.[40,99,100] Even in the phacoemulsification era, there is evidence to suggest that extended, complicated cases are at greater risk for progression (Figure 5-6).[80]

Since the introduction of phacoemulsification, studies evaluating the role of cataract surgery on the progression of diabetic retinopathy have reported variable and often contradictory results. Some authors have reported increased retinopathy progression,[99,101,102] whereas others have found no significant difference in the rate of progression after phacoemulsification when compared to fellow nonoperative eyes.[7,36,38,90] These varying results may be attributable to differences in baseline characteristics of the sample populations as well as variability in study design and data collection. The findings may also reflect the complexity of the disease itself and emphasize the point that progression of retinopathy is most often the result of multiple systemic and ocular factors.

cases where it is unclear whether the edema is Irvine-Gass or diabetic macular edema, it is reasonable to delay laser treatment for 3 to 6 months and first treat with topical NSAIDs and topical steroids to allow for regression of the Irvine-Gass component. If thickening persists beyond this period, presumption of a diabetic component is reasonable and intervention with laser therapy and/or intravitreal anti-VEGF or steroid injections may be appropriate. Progression of CSME/CME and response to therapy can be monitored with OCT in the postoperative period. It should be noted that anatomic success noted on OCT with resolution of thickening does not always correspond to visual improvement.[94]

PROGRESSION OF DIABETIC RETINOPATHY

Historically, there has been significant debate regarding progression of diabetic retinopathy after cataract surgery. Earlier studies demonstrated an increased incidence of NVI, neovascular glaucoma, vitreous hemorrhage, and progression of retinopathy after cataract surgery, particularly after ICCE.[95-97] Some authors reported progression of retinopathy after ECCE.[43,98,99] Others found no difference in the progression of retinopathy in the operated eyes and fellow nonoperative eyes.[41] Over the past 2 decades, cataract surgery has shifted from ICCE and ECCE to phacoemulsification.

SUMMARY

Cataracts are a significant cause of visual impairment among patients with diabetes. In the past, surgery for these patients was often deferred until vision was severely affected by the cataracts because of the significant risk for postoperative complications and vision loss. Today, advancement in the technique of cataract surgery has greatly improved the visual prognosis for patients with diabetes undergoing cataract surgery. Similarly, the perioperative implementation of laser therapy has greatly improved the visual potential in patients with diabetic retinopathy. Newer diagnostic modalities, such as OCT, and intravitreal injections of anti-VEGF agents and steroids have enhanced the outcome for successful cataract surgery in patients with diabetes.

The evolution of cataract surgery in patients with diabetes has moved from a risky undertaking with questionable results to a routine procedure with promising outcomes.

ACKNOWLEDGMENTS

The authors would like to acknowledge Dr. Jerry D. Cavallerano for his expertise and editorial skills and Robert Cavicchi for his help in acquiring fundus photographs and fluorescein angiograms.

Figure 5-6. Percentage of eyes with progression of diabetic retinopathy after ICCE versus ECCE (meta-analysis of available literature) versus phacoemulsification (unpublished Joslin data). (Reprinted with permission of Joslin Clinic, Boston, MA.)

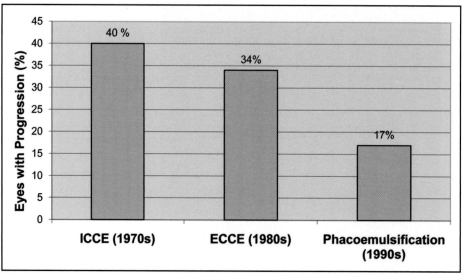

REFERENCES

1. IDF Diabetes Atlas. Global burden: prevalence and projections, 2010 and 2030. International Diabetes Federation Web site. http://www.diabetesatlas.org/content/diabetes-and-impaired-glucose-tolerance. Accessed December 7, 2009.
2. Klein R, Lee KE, Gangnon RE, Klein BE. The 25-year incidence of visual impairment in type 1 diabetes mellitus. The Wisconsin Epidemiologic Study of Diabetic Retinopathy. *Ophthalmology.* 2010;117:63-70.
3. Klein BE, Klein R, Moss SE. Incidence of cataract surgery in the Wisconsin Epidemiologic Study of Diabetic Retinopathy. *Am J Ophthalmol.* 1995;119:295-300.
4. Klein BE, Klein R, Moss SE. Prevalence of cataracts in a population-based study of persons with diabetes mellitus. *Ophthalmology.* 1985;92:1191-1196.
5. Klein BE, Klein R, Lee KE. Diabetes, cardiovascular disease, selected cardiovascular disease risk factors, and the 5-year incidence of age-related cataract and progression of lens opacities: the Beaver Dam Eye Study. *Am J Ophthalmol.* 1998;126:782-790.
6. Ederer F, Hiller R, Taylor HR. Senile lens changes and diabetes in two population studies. *Am J Ophthalmol.* 1981;91:381-395.
7. Chew EY, Benson WE, Remaley NA, et al. Results after lens extraction in patients with diabetic retinopathy: early treatment diabetic retinopathy study report number 25. *Arch Ophthalmol.* 1999;117:1600-1606.
8. Fintak DR, Ho AC. Perioperative and operative considerations in diabetics. *Ophthalmol Clin North Am.* 2006;19:427-434.
9. Podgor MJ, Kannel WB, Cassel GH, Sperduto RD. Lens changes and the incidence of cardiovascular events among persons with diabetes. *Am Heart J.* 1989;117:642-648.
10. Kador PF, Kinoshita JH. Diabetic and galactosaemic cataracts. *Ciba Found Symp.* 1984;106:110-131.
11. Kinoshita JH, Fukushi S, Kador P, Merola LO. Aldose reductase in diabetic complications of the eye. *Metabolism.* 1979;28:462-469.
12. Duke-Elder WS. Changes in refraction in diabetes mellitus. *Br J Ophthalmol.* 1925;9:167-187.
13. Okamoto F, Sone H, Nonoyama T, Hommura S. Refractive changes in diabetic patients during intensive glycaemic control. *Br J Ophthalmol.* 2000;84:1097-1102.
14. Blankenship GW, Machemer R. Long-term diabetic vitrectomy results. Report of 10 year follow-up. *Ophthalmology.* 1985;92:503-506.
15. Novak MA, Rice TA, Michels RG, Auer C. The crystalline lens after vitrectomy for diabetic retinopathy. *Ophthalmology.* 1984;91:1480-1484.
16. Holekamp NM, Shui YB, Beebe DC. Vitrectomy surgery increases oxygen exposure to the lens: a possible mechanism for nuclear cataract formation. *Am J Ophthalmol.* 2005;139:302-310.
17. Smiddy WE, Feuer W. Incidence of cataract extraction after diabetic vitrectomy. *Retina.* 2004;24:574-581.
18. Holekamp NM, Shui YB, Beebe D. Lower intraocular oxygen tension in diabetic patients: possible contribution to decreased incidence of nuclear sclerotic cataract. *Am J Ophthalmol.* 2006;141:1027-1032.
19. Wilson ME Jr, Levin AV, Trivedi RH, et al. Cataract associated with type-1 diabetes mellitus in the pediatric population. *J AAPOS.* 2007;11:162-165.
20. Datta V, Swift PG, Woodruff GH, Harris RF. Metabolic cataracts in newly diagnosed diabetes. *Arch Dis Child.* 1997;76:118-120.
21. Datiles MB III, Kador PF. Type I diabetic cataract. *Arch Ophthalmol.* 1999;117:284-285.
22. Falck A, Laatikainen L. Diabetic cataract in children. *Acta Ophthalmol Scand.* 1998;76:238-240.
23. Dickey JB, Daily MJ. Transient posterior subcapsular lens opacities in diabetes mellitus. *Am J Ophthalmol.* 1993;115:234-238.
24. Sanz S, Lillo J, Arruga J. Reversibility of cataracts in diabetes. *Scientific World Journal.* 2008;8:1148-1149.
25. Risk factors associated with age-related nuclear and cortical cataract: a case-control study in the Age-Related Eye Disease Study, AREDS Report No. 5. *Ophthalmology.* 2001;108:1400-1408.
26. Leske MC, Chylack LT Jr, Wu SY. The Lens Opacities Case-Control Study. Risk factors for cataract. *Arch Ophthalmol.* 1991;109:244-251.
27. Hiller R, Sperduto RD, Ederer F. Epidemiologic associations with nuclear, cortical, and posterior subcapsular cataracts. *Am J Epidemiol.* 1986;124:916-925.
28. Edwards MG, Schachat AP, Bressler SB, Bressler NM. Outcome of cataract operations performed to permit diagnosis, to determine eligibility for laser therapy, or to perform laser therapy of retinal disorders. *Am J Ophthalmol.* 1994;118:440-444.

29. Murtha T, Cavallerano J. The management of diabetic eye disease in the setting of cataract surgery. *Curr Opin Ophthalmol.* 2007;18:13-18.

30. Somaiya MD, Burns JD, Mintz R, Warren RE, Uchida T, Godley BF. Factors affecting visual outcomes after small-incision phacoemulsification in diabetic patients. *J Cataract Refract Surg.* 2002;28:1364-1371.

31. Pollack A, Leiba H, Bukelman A, Oliver M. Cystoid macular oedema following cataract extraction in patients with diabetes. *Br J Ophthalmol.* 1992;76:221-224.

32. Kirmani TH. Prognosis of cataract extraction in diabetics. *Am J Ophthalmol.* 1964;57:617-619.

33. Caird FI, Hutchinson M, Pirie A. Cataract extraction and diabetes. *Br J Ophthalmol.* 1965;49:466-471.

34. Benson WE, Brown GC, Tasman W, McNamara JA, Vander JF. Extracapsular cataract extraction with placement of a posterior chamber lens in patients with diabetic retinopathy. *Ophthalmology.* 1993;100:730-738.

35. Schatz H, Atienza D, McDonald HR, Johnson RN. Severe diabetic retinopathy after cataract surgery. *Am J Ophthalmol.* 1994;117:314-321.

36. Krepler K, Biowski R, Schrey S, Jandrasits K, Wedrich A. Cataract surgery in patients with diabetic retinopathy: visual outcome, progression of diabetic retinopathy, and incidence of diabetic macular oedema. *Graefes Arch Clin Exp Ophthalmol.* 2002;240:735-738.

37. Mittra RA, Borrillo JL, Dev S, Mieler WF, Koenig SB. Retinopathy progression and visual outcomes after phacoemulsification in patients with diabetes mellitus. *Arch Ophthalmol.* 2000;118:912-917.

38. Squirrell D, Bhola R, Bush J, Winder S, Talbot JF. A prospective, case controlled study of the natural history of diabetic retinopathy and maculopathy after uncomplicated phacoemulsification cataract surgery in patients with type 2 diabetes. *Br J Ophthalmol.* 2002;86:565-571.

39. Dowler JG, Sehmi KS, Hykin PG, Hamilton AM. The natural history of macular edema after cataract surgery in diabetes. *Ophthalmology.* 1999;106:663-668.

40. Dowler JG, Hykin PG, Hamilton AM. Phacoemulsification versus extracapsular cataract extraction in patients with diabetes. *Ophthalmology.* 2000;107:457-462.

41. Henricsson M, Heijl A, Janzon L. Diabetic retinopathy before and after cataract surgery. *Br J Ophthalmol.* 1996;80:789-793.

42. Dowler JG, Hykin PG, Lightman SL, Hamilton AM. Visual acuity following extracapsular cataract extraction in diabetes: a meta-analysis. *Eye (Lond).* 1995;9:313-317.

43. Pollack A, Leiba H, Bukelman A, Abrahami S, Oliver M. The course of diabetic retinopathy following cataract surgery in eyes previously treated by laser photocoagulation. *Br J Ophthalmol.* 1992;76:228-231.

44. Hykin PG, Gregson RM, Stevens JD, Hamilton PA. Extracapsular cataract extraction in proliferative diabetic retinopathy. *Ophthalmology.* 1993;100:394-399.

45. Cunliffe IA, Flanagan DW, George ND, Aggarwaal RJ, Moore AT. Extracapsular cataract surgery with lens implantation in diabetics with and without proliferative retinopathy. *Br J Ophthalmol.* 1991;75:9-12.

46. Schein OD, Katz J, Bass EB, et al. The value of routine preoperative medical testing before cataract surgery. Study of Medical Testing for Cataract Surgery. *N Engl J Med.* 2000;342:168-175.

47. Keay L, Lindsley K, Tielsch J, Katz J, Schein O. Routine preoperative medical testing for cataract surgery. *Cochrane Database Syst Rev.* 2009;CD007293.

48. Nascimento MA, Lira RP, Soares PH, Spessatto N, Kara-Jose N, Arieta CE. Are routine preoperative medical tests needed with cataract surgery? Study of visual acuity outcome. *Curr Eye Res.* 2004;28:285-290.

49. Elman MJ, Aiello LP, Beck RW, et al. Randomized trial evaluating ranibizumab plus prompt or deferred laser or triamcinolone plus prompt laser for diabetic macular edema. *Ophthalmology.* 2010;117:1064-1077.

50. Lanzagorta-Aresti A, Palacios-Pozo E, Menezo Rozalen JL, Navea-Tejerina A. Prevention of vision loss after cataract surgery in diabetic macular edema with intravitreal bevacizumab: a pilot study. *Retina.* 2009;29:530-535.

51. Akinci A, Batman C, Ozkilic E, Altinsoy A. Phacoemulsification with intravitreal bevacizumab injection in diabetic patients with macular edema and cataract. *Retina.* 2009;29:1432-1435.

52. Lam DS, Chan CK, Mohamed S, et al. Phacoemulsification with intravitreal triamcinolone in patients with cataract and coexisting diabetic macular oedema: a 6-month prospective pilot study. *Eye (Lond).* 2005;19:885-890.

53. Habib MS, Cannon PS, Steel DH. The combination of intravitreal triamcinolone and phacoemulsification surgery in patients with diabetic foveal oedema and cataract. *BMC Ophthalmol.* 2005;5:15.

54. Beck RW, Edwards AR, Aiello LP, et al. Three-year follow-up of a randomized trial comparing focal/grid photocoagulation and intravitreal triamcinolone for diabetic macular edema. *Arch Ophthalmol.* 2009;127:245-251.

55. Donnenfeld ED, Perry HD, Wittpenn JR, Solomon R, Nattis A, Chou T. Preoperative ketorolac tromethamine 0.4% in phacoemulsification outcomes: pharmacokinetic-response curve. *J Cataract Refract Surg.* 2006;32:1474-1482.

56. Krepler K, Ries E, Derbolav A, Nepp J, Wedrich A. Inflammation after phacoemulsification in diabetic retinopathy. Foldable acrylic versus heparin-surface-modified poly(methyl methacrylate) intraocular lenses. *J Cataract Refract Surg.* 2001;27:233-238.

57. Gatinel D, Lebrun T, Le Toumelin P, Chaine G. Aqueous flare induced by heparin-surface-modified poly(methyl methacrylate) and acrylic lenses implanted through the same-size incision in patients with diabetes. *J Cataract Refract Surg.* 2001;27:855-860.

58. Tewari A, Shah GK. Presbyopia-correcting intraocular lenses: what retinal surgeons should know. *Retina.* 2008;28:535-537.

59. Cillino S, Casuccio A, Di Pace F, et al. One-year outcomes with new-generation multifocal intraocular lenses. *Ophthalmology.* 2008;115:1508-1516.

60. Kamath GG, Prasad S, Danson A, Phillips RP. Visual outcome with the array multifocal intraocular lens in patients with concurrent eye disease. *J Cataract Refract Surg.* 2000;26:576-581.

61. Zeng M, Liu Y, Liu X, et al. Aberration and contrast sensitivity comparison of aspherical and monofocal and multifocal intraocular lens eyes. *Clin Experiment Ophthalmol.* 2007;35:355-360.

62. Zhao G, Zhang J, Zhou Y, Hu L, Che C, Jiang N. Visual function after monocular implantation of apodized diffractive multifocal or single-piece monofocal intraocular lens Randomized prospective comparison. *J Cataract Refract Surg.* 2010;36:282-285.

63. Kohnen T, Allen D, Boureau C, et al. European multicenter study of the AcrySof ReSTOR apodized diffractive intraocular lens. *Ophthalmology.* 2006;113:584.

64. Regan D, Neima D. Low-contrast letter charts in early diabetic retinopathy, ocular hypertension, glaucoma, and Parkinson's disease. *Br J Ophthalmol.* 1984;68:885-889.

65. Rodriguez-Galietero A, Montes-Mico R, Munoz G, Albarran-Diego C. Blue-light filtering intraocular lens in patients with diabetes: contrast sensitivity and chromatic discrimination. *J Cataract Refract Surg.* 2005;31:2088-2092.

66. Caporossi A, Casprini F, Martone G, Balestrazzi A, Tosi GM, Ciompi L. Contrast sensitivity evaluation of aspheric and spherical intraocular lenses 2 years after implantation. *J Refract Surg.* 2009;25:578-590.

67. Trueb PR, Albach C, Montes-Mico R, Ferrer-Blasco T. Visual acuity and contrast sensitivity in eyes implanted with aspheric and spherical intraocular lenses. *Ophthalmology.* 2009;116:890-895.

68. Chung TY, Chung H, Lee JH. Combined surgery and sequential surgery comprising phacoemulsification, pars plana vitrectomy, and intraocular lens implantation: comparison of clinical outcomes. *J Cataract Refract Surg.* 2002;28:2001-2005.

69. Lahey JM, Francis RR, Kearney JJ. Combining phacoemulsification with pars plana vitrectomy in patients with proliferative diabetic retinopathy: a series of 223 cases. *Ophthalmology.* 2003;110:1335-1339.

70. Diolaiuti S, Senn P, Schmid MK, Job O, Maloca P, Schipper I. Combined pars plana vitrectomy and phacoemulsification with intraocular lens implantation in severe proliferative diabetic retinopathy. *Ophthalmic Surg Lasers Imaging.* 2006;37:468-474.

71. Koenig SB, Mieler WF, Han DP, Abrams GW. Combined phacoemulsification, pars plana vitrectomy, and posterior chamber intraocular lens insertion. *Arch Ophthalmol.* 1992;110:1101-1104.

72. Sneed S, Parrish RK, Mandelbaum S, O'Grady G. Technical problems of extracapsular cataract extractions after vitrectomy. *Arch Ophthalmol.* 1986;104:1126-1127.

73. Smiddy WE, Stark WJ, Michels RG, Maumenee AE, Terry AC, Glaser BM. Cataract extraction after vitrectomy. *Ophthalmology.* 1987;94:483-487.

74. Hurley C, Barry P. Combined endocapsular phacoemulsification, pars plana vitrectomy, and intraocular lens implantation. *J Cataract Refract Surg.* 1996;22:462-466.

75. Blankenship GW, Flynn HW Jr, Kokame GT. Posterior chamber intraocular lens insertion during pars plana lensectomy and vitrectomy for complications of proliferative diabetic retinopathy. *Am J Ophthalmol.* 1989;108:1-5.

76. Zaczek A, Olivestedt G, Zetterstrom C. Visual outcome after phacoemulsification and IOL implantation in diabetic patients. *Br J Ophthalmol.* 1999;83:1036-1041.

77. Mirza SA, Alexandridou A, Marshall T, Stavrou P. Surgically induced miosis during phacoemulsification in patients with diabetes mellitus. *Eye (Lond).* 2003;17:194-199.

78. Smith SA, Smith SE. Evidence for a neuropathic aetiology in the small pupil of diabetes mellitus. *Br J Ophthalmol.* 1983;67:89-93.

79. Fujii T, Ishikawa S, Uga S. Ultrastructure of iris muscles in diabetes mellitus. *Ophthalmologica.* 1977;174:228-239.

80. Dev S, Pulido JS, Tessler HH, Mittra RA, Han DP, Mieler WF, Connor TB, Jr. Progression of diabetic retinopathy after endophthalmitis. *Ophthalmology.* 1999;106:774-781.

81. Phillips WB, Tasman WS. Postoperative endophthalmitis in association with diabetes mellitus. *Ophthalmology.* 1994;101:508-518.

82. Doft BH, Wisniewski SR, Kelsey SF, Fitzgerald SG. Diabetes and postoperative endophthalmitis in the endophthalmitis vitrectomy study. *Arch Ophthalmol.* 2001;119:650-656.

83. Ebihara Y, Kato S, Oshika T, Yoshizaki M, Sugita G. Posterior capsule opacification after cataract surgery in patients with diabetes mellitus. *J Cataract Refract Surg.* 2006;32:1184-1187.

84. Hayashi K, Hayashi H, Nakao F, Hayashi F. Posterior capsule opacification after cataract surgery in patients with diabetes mellitus. *Am J Ophthalmol.* 2002;134:10-16.

85. Kato S, Oshika T, Numaga J, et al. Anterior capsular contraction after cataract surgery in eyes of diabetic patients. *Br J Ophthalmol.* 2001;85:21-23.

86. Hayashi H, Hayashi K, Nakao F, Hayashi F. Area reduction in the anterior capsule opening in eyes of diabetes mellitus patients. *J Cataract Refract Surg.* 1998;24:1105-1110.

87. Wakabayashi T, Oshima Y, Sakaguchi H, et al. Intravitreal bevacizumab to treat iris neovascularization and neovascular glaucoma secondary to ischemic retinal diseases in 41 consecutive cases. *Ophthalmology.* 2008;115:1571-80, 1580.

88. Avery RL, Pearlman J, Pieramici DJ, et al. Intravitreal bevacizumab (Avastin) in the treatment of proliferative diabetic retinopathy. *Ophthalmology.* 2006;113:1695-15.

89. Avery RL. Regression of retinal and iris neovascularization after intravitreal bevacizumab (Avastin) treatment. *Retina.* 2006;26:352-354.

90. Romero-Aroca P, Fernandez-Ballart J, Almena-Garcia M, Mendez-Marin I, Salvat-Serra M, Buil-Calvo JA. Nonproliferative diabetic retinopathy and macular edema progression after phacoemulsification: prospective study. *J Cataract Refract Surg.* 2006;32:1438-1444.

91. Kim SJ, Equi R, Bressler NM. Analysis of macular edema after cataract surgery in patients with diabetes using optical coherence tomography. *Ophthalmology.* 2007;114:881-889.

92. Gass JD, Norton EW. Cystoid macular edema and papilledema following cataract extraction. A fluorescein fundoscopic and angiographic study. *Arch Ophthalmol.* 1966;76:646-661.

93. Photocoagulation for diabetic macular edema. Early Treatment Diabetic Retinopathy Study report number 1. Early Treatment Diabetic Retinopathy Study research group. *Arch Ophthalmol.* 1985;103:1796-1806.

94. Browning DJ, Glassman AR, Aiello LP, et al. Relationship between optical coherence tomography-measured central retinal thickness and visual acuity in diabetic macular edema. *Ophthalmology.* 2007;114:525-536.

95. Aiello LM, Wand M, Liang G. Neovascular glaucoma and vitreous hemorrhage following cataract surgery in patients with diabetes mellitus. *Ophthalmology.* 1983;90:814-820.

96. Poliner LS, Christianson DJ, Escoffery RF, Kolker AE, Gordon ME. Neovascular glaucoma after intracapsular and extracapsular cataract extraction in diabetic patients. *Am J Ophthalmol.* 1985;100:637-643.

97. Pollack A, Dotan S, Oliver M. Course of diabetic retinopathy following cataract surgery. *Br J Ophthalmol.* 1991;75:2-8.

98. Jaffe GJ, Burton TC, Kuhn E, Prescott A, Hartz A. Progression of nonproliferative diabetic retinopathy and visual outcome after extracapsular cataract extraction and intraocular lens implantation. *Am J Ophthalmol.* 1992;114:448-456.

99. Sadiq SA, Sleep T, Amoaku WM. The visual results and changes in retinopathy in diabetic patients following cataract surgery. *Eur J Ophthalmol.* 1999;9:14-20.

100. Antcliff RJ, Poulson A, Flanagan DW. Phacoemulsification in diabetics. *Eye (Lond).* 1996;10:737-741.

101. Hong T, Mitchell P, de Loryn T, Rochtchina E, Cugati S, Wang JJ. Development and progression of diabetic retinopathy 12 months after phacoemulsification cataract surgery. *Ophthalmology.* 2009;116:1510-1514.

102. Chung J, Kim MY, Kim HS, Yoo JS, Lee YC. Effect of cataract surgery on the progression of diabetic retinopathy. *J Cataract Refract Surg.* 2002;28:626-630.

6

Diabetes Mellitus and Optic Nerve Abnormalities

Jesse Richman, MD; King To, MD; Larissa Camejo, MD; and Alejandro Espaillat, MD

The optic nerve is formed by 1.0 to 1.5 million retinal ganglion cell axons and transmits visual information to the occipital cortex. The optic nerve is approximately 50 mm in length from the eye to the optic chiasm. Development of the optic nerve begins during the 6th week of gestation with ganglion cell axons entering the embryonic optic stalk. The intraocular segment of the optic nerve, which is visible on ophthalmic examination, is termed the *optic disc* or *optic nerve head* (Figure 6-1). The optic disc measures 1.5 mm horizontally and 1.75 mm vertically. Within the center of the optic disc is a depression termed the *physiologic cup*. The optic nerve head can be divided into superficial, prelaminar, laminar, and postlaminar portions.

Many diseases of the optic nerve head occur because of its anatomy and vascular supply. Axons of the retinal ganglion cells travel across the retina within the nerve fiber layer. The nerve fibers course toward the scleral canal to form the optic nerve in either a straight or arcuate fashion, depending on its originating location. The nerve fiber layer relies on axonal transport of metabolic products. Interruption of axonal transport at the optic disc from ischemia or inflammation results in optic disc edema.

Blood supply to the optic nerve comes from the central retinal artery and the posterior ciliary arteries, both branches of the ophthalmic artery (Figure 6-2). The superficial nerve fiber layer is supplied by the central

retinal artery. The prelaminar and laminar portions are supplied by the short posterior ciliary arteries (branches of the posterior ciliary arteries) and by the circle of Zinn-Haller, when it exists. The retrolaminar portion is supplied by short posterior ciliary arteries and pial arterial branches. Tissue whose vasculature is supplied by the short posterior ciliary arteries is susceptible to ischemia because these vessels are end arterioles.

ACUTE OPTIC DISC EDEMA

Diabetic Papillopathy

Diabetic papillopathy is a rare optic nerve condition originally described by Lubow and Makley in young patients with type 1 diabetes.[1,2] The pathophysiology is presumed to be due to mild, usually reversible ischemia. However, the presentation is different from other ischemic conditions of the optic nerve head, such as nonarteritic anterior ischemic optic neuropathy. Patients typically present asymptomatically or with nonpainful, mild blurring of their vision. Involvement can be unilateral or bilateral. Visual acuity can be normal or slightly reduced. Fundus examination reveals a hyperemic and edematous optic disc with little if any diabetic retinopathy (Figure 6-3). The dilated, radially oriented,

Espaillat A.
Diabetic Eye Disease: A Comprehensive Review (pp. 41-48)
© 2012 SLACK Incorporated

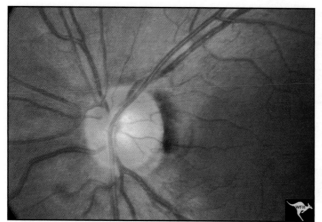

Figure 6-1. Normal optic disc. (Reproduced with permission from Hoyt WF. "IIB1_01a:Normal peripapillary nerve fiber layer." Neuro-Ophthalmology Virtual Education Library: NOVEL. 2002. Online Image.)

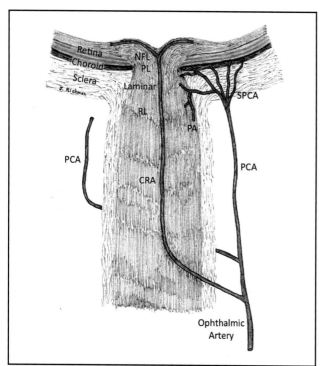

Figure 6-2. Blood flow to the anterior optic nerve. NFL = nerve fiber layer; PL = prelaminar; RL = retrolaminar; PA = pial arterial branches; SPCA = short posterior ciliary artery; PCA = posterior ciliary artery; CRA = central retinal artery. (Illustration by Jesse Richman, MD.)

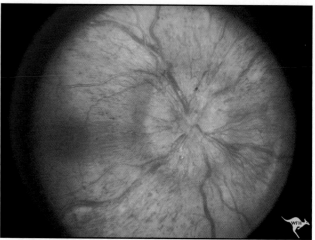

Figure 6-3. Diabetic papillopathy. (Reproduced with permission from Hoyt, William F. "B2_03:Disc swelling. Diabetic papillopathy" Neuro-Ophthalmology Virtual Education Library: NOVEL. 2002. Online Image.)

diffuse. Patients have little optic nerve dysfunction; normal intracranial pressure; and no inflammatory, infectious, or infiltrative process.

Although initially thought to be a manifestation of type 1 diabetes, multiple studies have described diabetic papillopathy in older patients with type 2 diabetes.[4,5] These patients may be more likely to have bilateral disease, duration of diabetes for more than 8 to 10 years, and varying degrees of diabetic retinopathy.[4,5] If patients have bilateral papillopathy, it is recommended to obtain magnetic resonance imaging (MRI) and lumbar puncture to rule out an intracranial mass or increased intracranial pressure. Diabetic papillopathy typically is self-limited, resolving within 2 to 10 months with no optic atrophy. Rarely, diabetic papillopathy may precede the development of anterior ischemic optic neuropathy. There is no proven therapy for diabetic papillopathy.

Nonarteritic Anterior Ischemic Optic Neuropathy

Nonarteritic anterior ischemic optic neuropathy (NAION) is caused by compromise to branches of the short posterior ciliary arteries. Experimental occlusion of the posterior ciliary arteries in monkeys has shown that the axons of the prelaminar nerve become swollen due to obstruction of axonal transport at the lamina cribrosa, and the laminar and retrolaminar portions show ischemic changes. Nocturnal hypotension may play a role in the pathogenesis of NAION due to lack of perfusion in watershed areas between the medial and lateral short posterior ciliary arteries. Decreased anastomotic blood flow from the central retinal artery to the prelaminar, laminar, and retrolaminar regions may be

telangiectatic vessels of the disc may resemble neovascularization; however, there is no leakage on fluorescein angiography (FA) and these vessels do not proliferate into the vitreous cavity. These prominent vessels disappear when the optic disc swelling resolves. Early phase of the FA shows no delay in filling of the choroid or the disc and the late phase shows hyperfluorescence of the disc.[3] Visual field testing may reveal minimal field loss or an enlarged blind spot if the optic disc edema is

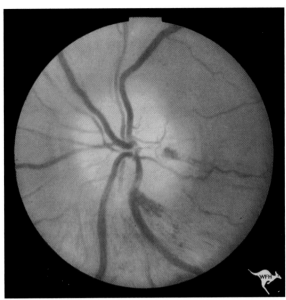

Figure 6-4. Non-arteritic anterior ischemic optic neuropathy. (Reproduced with permission from Hoyt, William F. "B1_05:Disc swelling. Ischemic papillopathies. AION" Neuro-Ophthalmology Virtual Education Library: NOVEL. 2002. Online Image.)

present due to aging, arteriolosclerosis, and atherosclerosis, making the tissue more susceptible to infarction.

Structural factors of the optic disc are important in the pathogenesis of NAION. Anatomical crowding of the optic disc, evidenced by a small or absent physiological cup, may predispose the disc to blockage of axonal flow or amplify ischemia. The optic disc in the fellow eye usually also has a small cup, which is useful in diagnosing NAION because the details of the cup may be obscured in an eye with a recent NAION. There is an increased frequency of upper disc involvement. It is rare to have repeat attacks in the same eye, although this may represent decompression of the nerve from focal optic nerve atrophy.[6]

Patients present with sudden visual loss over days to hours, often upon wakening in the morning, possibly related to systemic nocturnal hypotension. Patients have an afferent pupillary defect and a visual field defect (inferior altitudinal most common) with visual acuity ranging from 20/20 to no light perception at presentation. The optic disc typically shows pallid swelling, which may be diffuse or sectoral (Figure 6-4). There are often accompanying splinter hemorrhages and cotton wool spots. Fluorescein angiography may show delayed peripapillary choroidal filling, delayed retinal artery appearance time, increased retinal circulation time, and late staining of the disc. The edema typically resolves, leaving atrophy in the area of previous edema and focal attenuation of arterioles exiting the disc after 4 to 6 weeks. If optic disc edema persists beyond this point, alternative diagnoses should be explored.

Patients with NAION are typically older than 50 and commonly have systemic risk factors. Although hypertension is the leading associated factor, up to 25% of patients with NAION have diabetes.[7] Diabetic microvascular changes may affect the anterior portion of the optic nerve causing ischemia.[8] There is no difference in age when diabetics and nondiabetics develop NAION. Patients with diabetes who develop NAION have a higher prevalence of hypertension, ischemic heart disease, and transient ischemic attacks. No differences are observed between patients with diabetes and those without diabetes in presenting visual acuity, percent with improvement or worsening acuity, or acuity 6 months from onset of NAION. Diabetics have less severe visual field defect initially, no difference in the percent that have an improved or worsened visual field, and no difference in visual field defect 6 months from the onset of NAION. Diabetics average one additional week of optic disc edema prior to resolution. When patients develop NAION in the fellow eye, diabetics have a shorter time to involvement in the fellow eye compared with nondiabetics.[9]

There is some disagreement as to whether diabetic papillopathy may actually be a mild form of NAION in patients with diabetes. Diabetic papillopathy often has little or no physiologic cup, which is characteristic of NAION. Also, asymptomatic optic disc edema can occur in the early stages of NAION, which is similar to the presentation of diabetic papillopathy. However, diabetic papillopathy should be suspected if the patient remains asymptomatic, has simultaneous bilateral presentation, no optic disc pallor, visual field loss that is not inferior altitudinal, normal filling on FA, a longer duration of disc edema, or a normal or large physiologic cup in the fellow eye (Table 6-1). In patients with diabetes, irreversible ischemia to the optic nerve head leads to NAION, whereas reversible ischemia likely causes diabetic papillopathy.

There is no proven treatment for NAION. Vasodilators, anticoagulants, antiplatelet agents, diphenylhydantoin, norepinephrine, intraocular pressure-lowering agents, and hyperbaric oxygen are not effective. The Ischemic Optic Neuropathy Decompression Trial showed that optic nerve sheath decompression improves the condition. The use of levodopa and corticosteroids is controversial. There is some evidence that aspirin may be beneficial in preventing the fellow eye from developing the condition.[10-12] There is a 15% 5-year risk and a 30% to 40% lifetime risk of development in the subsequent eye. Visual disability usually is stable due to the stable visual field defect.[13] Twenty-four months after NAION occurs, 31% improve ≥3 lines of visual acuity, 21.8% lose ≥3 lines of visual acuity, and the majority have stable visual acuity.[14]

Table 6-1. Comparison of Nonarteritic Anterior Ischemic Optic Neuropathy (NAION) and Diabetic Papillopathy

	NAION	*Diabetic Papillopathy*
Age	Older than 50	Any age (typically younger)
Presentation	Acute	Mild or asymptomatic
Optic disc appearance	Pallor or hyperemia	Hyperemic
Visual field	Altitudinal defect	Enlarged blind spot
Fluorescein angiography	Delayed filling of disc	Normal filling
Prognosis	Majority with stable defect	Resolution in 2 to 10 months

Optic Atrophy

Panretinal Photocoagulation

Pallor of the optic disc can occur after panretinal photocoagulation (PRP) or following spontaneous regression of proliferative retinopathy. Eyes that have received PRP can appear to have a glaucomatous appearance.[15] The glaucomatous appearance is due to areas of disc pallor corresponding to retinal nerve fiber layer (RNFL) loss, not increased cupping.[16-18] Optic disc cupping is not a feature of diabetes, despite both diabetes and glaucoma causing RNFL loss.[17]

Patients with diabetes have been shown to have a thinner RNFL than patients without diabetes.[19] The loss of ganglion cells and RNFL correlates with the severity of diabetic retinopathy.[20] Patients with diabetes who have had PRP have a thinner RNFL than those who have not undergone PRP.[16,21] Thinning of the RNFL may be due to the effects of PRP itself or more severe retinal ischemia. With the incidence of diabetes increasing and with the increasing popularity of devices that image the RNFL for the detection of glaucoma, caution must be used because patients with diabetes with or without a history of PRP have a thinner RNFL, which is not necessarily due to glaucoma.

Wolfram Syndrome

In 1938, Wolfram first reported a family in which 4 siblings had diabetes mellitus and optic atrophy, some of whom later developed hearing loss and a neurogenic bladder.[22] Wolfram syndrome is a neurodegenerative disorder characterized by diabetes insipidus, diabetes mellitus, optic atrophy, and deafness (a combination also known as DIDMOAD). The inheritance is autosomal recessive, affecting 1 in 500,000 to 770,000.[23] A variety of mutations of the WFS1 gene (4p16.1) and the CISD2 gene (4q22-q24) are associated with the syndrome. The WFS1 gene is responsible for most cases, with mutations of the CISD2 gene occurring in a few consanguineous families. The WFS1 gene code is for wolframin, a membrane glycoprotein in the endoplasmic reticulum that has a role in calcium channel trafficking and β-cell apoptosis in the pancreas and limbic system.[24,25]

Patients present in the first decade of life with diabetes mellitus and optic atrophy, which are essential components for diagnosing this syndrome. Diabetes mellitus typically presents at a median age of 6 years and optic atrophy at a median age of 11 years. The degree of atrophy is uniformly severe and progressive. Decreased visual acuity, constriction of visual fields, central scotomas, color vision defects, and cataract may be seen in addition to optic atrophy.[26] Most patients experience a reduction in vision to counting fingers after a median of 8 years. Diabetic retinopathy is rarely observed. Microvascular changes are not as common as those seen in patients with type 1 diabetes.[27]

Diabetes insipidus and deafness occur in the second decade; urinary tract abnormalities such as dilated renal outflow tracts and bladder atony occur in the third decade; and multiple neurological abnormalities such as seizures, ataxia, reduced reflexes, horizontal nystagmus, and peripheral neuropathy occur in the fourth decade.[28] MRI of the brain commonly shows reduced signal from the hypothalamus and pituitary, as well as generalized atrophy, especially in the cerebellum, medulla, and pons.[29] No correlation exists between the degree of bladder dysfunction and the degree of other abnormalities. Psychiatric manifestations may be prominent with severe depression, psychosis, and compulsive aggressiveness. The prognosis of patients with Wolfram syndrome is poor, with most patients dying at a median age of 30 years due to renal failure or respiratory failure from brainstem atrophy.

SUPERIOR SEGMENTAL OPTIC NERVE HYPOPLASIA

Superior segmental optic nerve hypoplasia is a rare condition affecting the superior portion of the optic nerve in the offspring of mothers with type 1 diabetes.[30,31] The exact pathogenesis is unclear, but it is bilateral in two-thirds of cases and affects females in three-fourths of cases.[32] The condition was first described by Petersen and Walton and has 4 characteristic features[33]:

1. Relative superior entrance of the central retinal artery
2. Pallor of the superior disc
3. Superior peripapillary halo
4. Thinning of the superior peripapillary nerve fiber layer (Figure 6-5)

Patients are typically asymptomatic, having normal visual acuity, normal color vision, and no systemic anomalies. Patients may also have generalized arteriolar tortuosity and an absent physiologic cup. Visual field testing reveals a stable inferior defect, which does not follow an arcuate pattern.[34,35] It has been hypothesized that this field pattern may represent direct damage to retinal ganglion cells.

A similar variant called topless optic disc syndrome has been described in Japan. It appears similar to superior segmental optic nerve hypoplasia but occurs in the absence of maternal diabetes.[36] Japanese patients with topless disc are born at term and have normal birth weight. Patients with superior segmental optic nerve hypoplasia may have short gestation time, low birth weight, and poor maternal diabetic control.[30] A detailed clinical examination and history are necessary to diagnose superior segmental optic nerve hypoplasia, obviating the need for further workup in these patients.

RELATIONSHIP BETWEEN DIABETES MELLITUS AND GLAUCOMA

Glaucoma is a leading cause of blindness.[37] It is a multifactorial condition, the risk factors of which are increasingly well defined from large-scale epidemiological studies. One risk factor that remains controversial is the presence of diabetes.[38] It has been proposed that diabetic eyes are at greater risk of injury from external stressors, such as elevated intraocular pressure.[39] Alternatively, diabetes may cause ganglion cell loss, which becomes additive to a glaucomatous ganglion cell injury. Several larger scale clinical trials, including

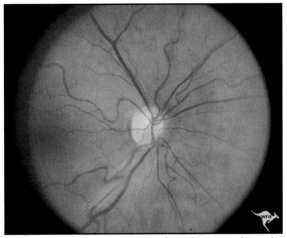

Figure 6-5. Superior segmental optic nerve hypoplasia. (Reproduced with permission from Hoyt, William F. "H_55:Superior segmental optic hypoplasia (SSOH). Topless disc syndrome" Neuro-Ophthalmology Virtual Education Library: NOVEL. 2002. Online Image.)

the Beaver Dam, Rotterdam, and Blue Mountains Eye studies, have reported an increased risk of open-angle glaucoma in people with diabetes.[40-42] However, no evidence for an association was reported in the Baltimore Eye Survey, the more recent Rotterdam Study, and the Framingham Eye Study.[43-45]

These studies showed inconsistencies probably due to a redefinition of primary open-angle glaucoma (POAG). A similar inconsistency has been identified by the authors of the Ocular Hypertension Treatment Study (OHTS). Initial multivariate analysis from the OHTS suggested that diabetes was protective against conversion from ocular hypertension to glaucoma; however, more recent analysis suggested that both the European Glaucoma Prevention study and the OHTS were underpowered to find an effect. The OHTS authors acknowledged that patient self-reporting of diabetes and their exclusion criteria may have produced a diabetic cohort that was atypical, leading to the observed protective outcome.[46-48]

As many of the above studies do not specifically set out to consider a link between diabetes and glaucoma, their selection and diagnostic criteria (self-report, glucose tolerance testing) differed substantially.[49] As such, the presence of opposing outcomes may not be surprising. The epidemiological evidence for an association between the 2 conditions remains inconclusive. There is a growing body of evidence that the presence of long-standing hyperglycemia, along with lipid abnormalities, may increase the risk of neuronal injury from stress.[49] Various pathways have been illustrated whereby diabetes and glaucoma might converge to produce an increased risk of neurodegeneration. These pathways can be summarized as follows[49]:

- Altered biochemical pathways compromise cells and also increase oxidative stress.
- Vascular changes can reduce blood flow and impair oxygen diffusion. Endothelial cell injury and dysfunction can reduce the capacity of auto-regulation to protect against fluctuations in eye and blood pressure, leading to relative hypoxia.
- Glial cell activation can lead to impaired ionic support and possibly reduced glutamate uptake, which might increase the chance of excitotoxicity. Excessive glial cell activation may also contribute to chronic inflammation.
- Changes to neurons may impair their ability to function, including axonal transport, leaving these neurons, which are already vulnerable, under additional stress.
- Connective tissue remodeling might reduce compliance at the trabecular meshwork and lamina cribrosa, promoting increased intraocular pressure and greater optic nerve head mechanical stress, respectively.

Further studies are needed to directly determine mechanisms underlying any potential association between diabetes and glaucoma.

ACKNOWLEDGMENT

Thank you to Dr. Michael J. Pokabla for contributing some references and ideas to this chapter.

REFERENCES

1. Lubow M, Makley TA Jr. Pseudopapilledema of juvenile diabetes mellitus. *Arch Ophthalmol.* 1971;85:417-422.
2. Appen RE, Chandra SR, Klein R, Myers FL. Diabetic papillopathy. *Am J Ophthalmol.* 1980;90:203-209.
3. Sato T, Fujikado T, Hosohata J, et al. Development of bilateral, nonarteritic anterior ischemic optic neuropathy in an eye with diabetic papillopathy. *Jpn N Ophthalmol.* 2004;48:158-162.
4. Bayraktar Z, Alacali N, Bayraktar S. Diabetic papillopathy in type II diabetic patients. *Retina.* 2002;22:752-758.
5. Regillo CD, Brown C, Savino PJ, et al. Diabetic papillopathy. Patient characteristics and fundus findings. *Arch Ophthalmol.* 1995;113:889-895.
6. Hamed LM, Purvin V, Rosenberg M. Recurrent anterior ischemic optic neuropathy in young adults. *J Clin Neuroophthalmol.* 1988;8:239-248.
7. Hayreh SS, Joos KM, Podhajsky PA, Long CR. Systemic diseases associated with nonarteritic anterior ischemic optic neuropathy. *Am J Ophthalmol.* 1994;118:766-80.
8. Flammer J, Orgül S, Costa VP, et al. The impact of ocular blood flow in glaucoma. *Prog Ret Eye Res.* 2002;21:359-393.
9. Hayreh SS, Zimmerman MB. Nonarteritis anterior ischemic optic neuropathy: clinical characteristics in diabetic patients versus nondiabetic patients. *Ophthalmology.* 2008;115:1818-1825.
10. Newman NJ, Scherer R, Langenberg P, et al; Ischemic Optic Neuropathy Decompression Trial Research Group. The fellow eye in NAION: report from the ischemic optic neuropathy decompression trial follow-up study. *Am J Ophthalmol.* 2002;134:317-328.
11. Salomon O, Huna-Baron R, Steinberg DM, et al. Role of aspirin in reducing the frequency of second eye involvement in patients with non-arteritic anterior ischaemic optic neuropathy. *Eye.* 1999;13:357-359.
12. Kupersmith MJ, Frohman L, Sanderson M, et al. Aspirin reduces the incidence of second eye NAION: a retrospective study. *J Neuroophthalmol.* 1997;17:250-253.
13. Scherer RW, Feldon SE, Levin L, et al; Ischemic Optic Neuropathy Decompression Trial Research Group. Visual fields at follow-up in the Ischemic Optic Neuropathy Decompression Trial: evaluation of change in pattern defect and severity over time. *Ophthalmology.* 2008;115:1809-1817.
14. Ischemic optic neuropathy decompression trial: twenty-four-month update. *Arch Ophthalmol.* 2000;118:793-798.
15. Johns KJ, Leonard-Martin T, Feman S. The effect of panretinal photocoagulation on optic nerve cupping. *Ophthalmology.* 1989;96:211-216.
16. Lim MC, Tanimoto SA, Furlani BA, et al. Effect of diabetic retinopathy and panretinal photocoagulation on retinal nerve fiber layer and optic nerve appearance. *Arch Ophthalmol.* 2009;127:857-862.
17. Klein BE, Moss SE, Magli YL, Klein R, Hoyer C, Johnson J. Optic disc cupping: prevalence findings from the WESDR. *Invest Ophthalmol Vis Sci.* 1989;30:304-309.
18. Königsreuther KA, Jonas JB. Optic disc morphology in diabetes mellitus. *Graefes Arch Clin Exp Ophthalmol.* 1995;233:200-204.
19. Takahashi H, Goto T, Shoji T, et al. Diabetes-associated retinal nerve fiber damage evaluated with scanning laser polarimetry. *Am J Ophthalmol.* 2006;142:88-94.
20. Chihara E, Matsuoka T, Ogura Y, Matsumura M. Retinal nerve fiber layer defect as an early manifestation of diabetic retinopathy. *Ophthalmology.* 1993;100:1147-1151.
21. Hsu SY, Chung CP. Evaluation of retinal nerve fiber layer thickness in diabetic retinopathy after panretinal photocoagulation. *Kaohsiung J Med Sci.* 2002;18:397-400.
22. Wolfram D, Wagener HP. Diabetes mellitus and simple optic atrophy among siblings: report of four cases. *Proc Staff Meet Mayo Clin.* 1938;13:715-718.
23. Barrett TG, Bundey SE. Wolfram (DIDMOAD) syndrome. *J Med Genet.* 1997;34:838-841.
24. Riggs AC, Bernal-Mizrachi E, Ohsugi M, et al. Mice conditionally lacking the Wolfram gene in pancreatic islet beta cells exhibit diabetes as a result of enhanced endoplasmic reticulum stress and apoptosis. *Diabetologia.* 2005;48:2313-2321.
25. d'Annunzio G, Minuto N, D'Amato E, et al. Wolfram syndrome (diabetes insipidus, diabetes, optic atrophy, and deafness): clinical and genetic study. *Diabetes Care.* 2008;31:1743-1745.
26. Castro FJ, Barrio J, Perena MF, et al. Uncommon ophthalmologic findings associated with Wolfram syndrome. *Acta Ophthalmol Scand.* 2000;78:118-119.
27. Kinsley BT, Swift M, Dumont RH, Swift RG. Morbidity and mortality in the Wolfram syndrome. *Diabetes Care.* 1995;18:1566-1570.

28. Barrett TG, Bundey SE, Macleod AF. Neurodegeneration and diabetes: UK nationwide study of Wolfram (DIDMOAD) syndrome. *Lancet.* 1995;346:1458-1463.

29. Rando TA, Horton JC, Layzer RB. Wolfram syndrome: evidence of a diffuse neurodegenerative disease by magnetic resonance imaging. *Neurology.* 1992;42:1220-1224.

30. Landau K, Bajka JD, Kirchschläger BM. Topless optic disks in children of mothers with type I diabetes mellitus. *Am J Ophthalmol.* 1998;125:605-611.

31. Takagi M, Abe H, Hatase T, et al. Superior segmental optic nerve hypoplasia in youth. *Jpn J Ophthalmol.* 2008;52:468-474.

32. Foroozan R. Superior segmental optic nerve hypoplasia and diabetes mellitus. *J Diabetes Complications.* 2005;19:165-167.

33. Peterson RA, Walton DS. Optic nerve hypoplasia with a good visual acuity and visual field defects. *Arch Ophthalmol.* 1977;95:254-258.

34. Hayashi K, Tomidokoro A, Aihara M, et al. Long-term follow-up of superior segmental optic hypoplasia. *Jpn J Ophthalmol.* 2008;52:412-414.

35. Kim RY, Hoyt WF, Lessell S, Narahara M. Superior segmental optic hypoplasia. *Arch Ophthalmol.* 1989;107:1312-1316.

36. Hashimoto M, Ohtsuka K, Nakagawa T, Hoyt WF. Topless optic disk syndrome without maternal diabetes mellitus. *Am J Ophthalmol.* 1999;128:111-112.

37. Quigley HA. Number of people with glaucoma worldwide. *Br J Ophthalmol.* 1996;80:389-393.

38. Quigley HA, Broman AT. The number of people with glaucoma worldwide in 2010 and 2020. *Br J Ophthalmol.* 2006;90:262-267.

39. Becker B. Diabetes mellitus and primary open angle glaucoma. The XXVII Edward Jackson Memorial Lecture. *Am J Ophthalmol.* 1971;1:1-16.

40. Klein BE, Klein R, Jensen SC. Open angle glaucoma and older onset diabetes. The Beaver Dam Eye Study. *Ophthalmology.* 1994;101:1173-1177.

41. Dielemans I, de Jong PT, Stolk R, Vingerling JR, Grobbee DE, Hofman A. Primary open angle glaucoma, intraocular pressure, and diabetes mellitus in the general elderly population. The Rotterdam Study. *Ophthalmology.* 1996;103:1271-1275.

42. Mitchell P, Smith W, Chey T, Healey PR. Open angle glaucoma and diabetes: the Blue Mountains eye study, Australia. *Ophthalmology.* 1997;104:712-718.

43. Tielsch JM, Katz J, Quigley HA, Javitt JC, Sommer A. Diabetes, intraocular pressure, and primary open-angle glaucoma in the Baltimore Eye Survey. *Ophthalmology.* 1995;102:48-53.

44. De Voogd S, Ikram MK, Wolfs RC, et al. Is diabetes mellitus a risk factor for open-angle glaucoma? The Rotterdam Study. *Ophthalmology.* 2006;113:1827-1831.

45. Kanh HA, Leibowitz HM, Ganley JP, et al. The Framingham Eye Study. II. Association of ophthalmic pathology with single variables previously measured in the Framingham Heart Study. *Am J Epidemiol.* 1977;106:33-41.

46. Gordon MO, Beiser JA, Brandt JD, et al. The Ocular Hypertension Treatment Study: baseline factors that predict the onset of primary open-angle glaucoma. *Arch Ophthalmol.* 2002;120:714-720.

47. Coleman AL, Miglior S. Risk factors for glaucoma onset and progression. *Surv Ophthalmol.* 2008;53(Suppl)1:S3-S10.

48. Gordon MO, Beiser JA, Kass MA. Is a history of diabetes mellitus protective against developing open-angle glaucoma? *Arch Ophthalmol.* 2008;126:280-281.

49. Wong V, Bui B, Vingrys A. Clinical and experimental links between diabetes and glaucoma. *Clin Experiment Optom.* 2011;94:4-23.

7

Diabetes Mellitus and Macular Abnormalities

Alejandro Espaillat, MD

INTRODUCTION

Diabetes affects approximately 20 million people in the United States, and roughly 10 times that number worldwide.[1] The prevalence of diabetes has tripled in the United States over the past 25 years and has increased rapidly throughout the rest of the world.[2] Experts foresee continued growth in the diabetic population, with projections that it will expand to include 439 million people by 2030.[3]

Visual impairment associated with diabetes mellitus and diabetic eye disease may result from diabetic macular edema, macular ischemia, vitreous hemorrhage, or diabetic tractional retinal detachment. Of all these causes, retinal edema, threatening or involving the macula, is an important visual consequence of abnormal retinal vascular permeability, and it is the most common cause of vision loss among patients with diabetes. Data from the Wisconsin Epidemiologic Study of Diabetic Retinopathy suggest that the 14-year incidence of diabetic macular edema is 26%.[4]

Definition

Diabetic macular edema is clinically seen as thickening of the retina. The Early Treatment Diabetic Retinopathy Study (ETDRS) was a randomized, prospective, clinical trial evaluating photocoagulation and aspirin treatment in patients with diabetes with less than high-risk proliferative diabetic retinopathy (PDR) in both eyes. The treatment outcome measurement in the ETDRS was moderate visual loss comparing baseline to follow-up visual acuities. Moderate visual loss was defined as doubling of the visual angle (eg, a decrease from 20/20 to 20/40 or from 20/50 to 20/100, a decrease of 15 or more letters on ETDRS visual acuity charts, or a loss of 3 or more lines of Snellen equivalent). The ETDRS has further classified diabetic macular edema to assist physicians in decision making regarding its treatment.[5-8]

The ETDRS defined clinically significant macular edema (CSME) as edema satisfying any 1 of the following 3 criteria: 1) any retinal thickening within 500 μm of the center of the macula (Figure 7-1); 2) hard exudates within 500 μm of the center of the macula with adjacent retinal thickening (Figure 7-2); or 3) retinal thickening at least 1 disc area in size, any part of which is within 1 disc diameter of the center of the macula (Figure 7-3). The definition was based on an analysis of stereo color fundus photographs by trained graders without the use of the terms *focal* or *diffuse* and was also used by clinicians using stereo slit-lamp biomicroscopy to determine whether laser treatment was indicated.

The terms *focal* and *diffuse* are used frequently to differentiate between 2 types of diabetic macular edema; however, these 2 terms have not been defined consistently in the literature.[9] Focal diabetic macular edema, defined in a variety of ways, has been reported to be more common than diffuse diabetic macular

Espaillat A.
Diabetic Eye Disease: A Comprehensive Review (pp. 49-72)
© 2012 SLACK Incorporated

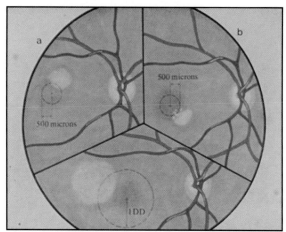

Figure 7-1. Retinal edema located at or within 500 µm of the center of the macula.

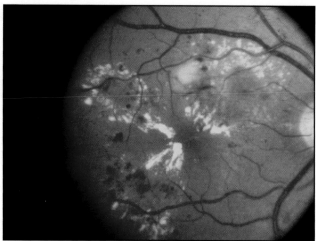

Figure 7-3. A zone of thickening larger than 1 disc area if located within 1 disc diameter of the center of the macula.

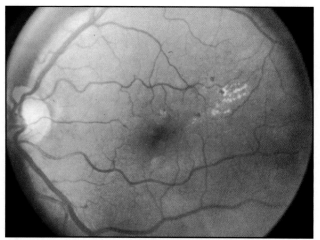

Figure 7-2. Hard exudates at or within 500 µm of the center if associated with thickening of adjacent retina.

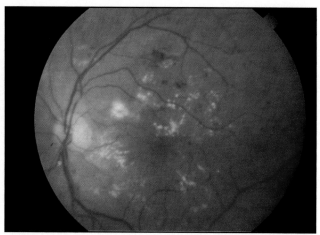

Figure 7-4. Two or more disc areas of retinal thickening involving the center of the macula.

edema; however, many cases of diabetic macular edema subjected to these definitions have mixed features, making a clear distinction difficult. Focal diabetic macular edema has been associated with less macular thickening, better visual acuity, and less severe retinopathy. Some authors have implied that the classification is predictive regarding outcomes after various treatments; however, the ETDRS, when defining the terms with respect to source of fluorescein leakage, did not support such a conclusion.

Others have contended that focal and diffuse diabetic macular edema differ in the need for fluorescein angiography as a guide in planning focal or grid laser treatment. A more frequent association of diffuse diabetic macular edema than focal diabetic macular edema is subretinal fibrosis and atrophic creep after macular laser photocoagulation. Critical evaluation of the evidence to support these assertions is important but hindered because the definition is often lacking or unclear. Additional confusion may ensue because the

term *focal* is used to describe a technique of applying laser directly to microaneurysms when treating diabetic macular edema with focal or grid photocoagulation. The published definitions for focal and diffuse diabetic macular edema have been based on 4 examination methods—fundus biomicroscopy, color fundus photography, fluorescein angiography, and optical coherence tomography (OCT).

Definitions involving color fundus photographs often involve area criteria. Diffuse macular edema has been defined as having 2 or more disc areas of retinal thickening with involvement of the center of the macula (Figure 7-4). Focal macular edema has been defined as an area of retinal thickening less than 2 disc areas in diameter not affecting the center of the macula (Figure 7-5).[10] Some authors imply that increased lipid exudates correlate with a more focal type of diabetic macular edema (Figure 7-6),[11] whereas others have defined edema in terms of having circinate rings of exudation (Figures 7-7). Definitions of diffuse and focal diabetic

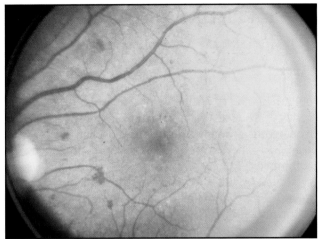

Figure 7-5. Area of retinal thickening less than 2 disc areas in diameter not affecting the center of the macula.

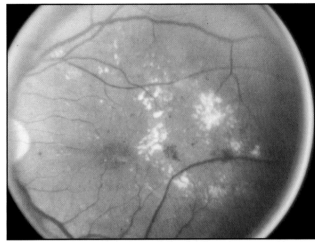

Figure 7-7. Other authors have defined edema in terms of having circinate rings of exudation adjacent to the center of macula.

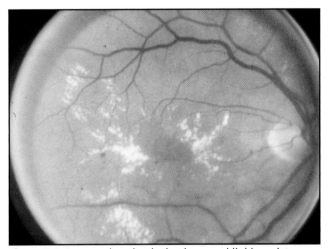

Figure 7-6. Some authors imply that increased lipid exudates correlate with a more focal type of diabetic macular edema.

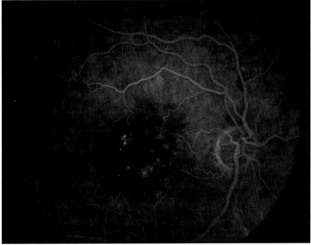

Figure 7-8. Fluorescein angiography showing cystoid spaces within the macula, filled with dye pooling in the late phase.

macular edema based on fluorescein angiography use cystoid macular edema as a criterion to categorize an eye as diffuse or focal (Figures 7-8).[12]

The use of OCT to define edema as focal or diffuse has been developed from 2 different perspectives—regional map and cross-sectional scans. In the false-color map, a sense of focality can be obtained when isolated islands of hot colors are surrounded by larger areas of cool colors, but this is difficult to quantitate. Using OCT, diffuse edema has been defined as thickened areas of lower reflectivity in the outer and inner retina but specifically without cystoid spaces, with retinal thickness exceeding 200 μm (Figure 7-9). No analogous definition of focal diabetic macular edema has been put forth. Definitions based on the morphological features of cross-sectional scans risk dependence on scanner technology. The Stratus OCT (Carl Zeiss Meditec, Dublin, CA) has finer resolution than the earlier versions with better ability to discriminate small cysts. Thus, eyes categorized as diffuse diabetic macular edema by the OCT 2 scanner (Carl Zeiss Meditec) may be categorized as having cysts by a Stratus OCT scanner and may be excluded from some definitions of diffuse diabetic macular edema.

Hybrid definitions have been used frequently to define diffuse diabetic macular edema but not focal diabetic macular edema. The definitions can be categorized into a subgroup using clinical examination and fluorescein angiography criteria and a subgroup using clinical examination, fluorescein angiography, and OCT criteria. Broadly speaking, the definitions differ in regard to how much of the macula must be thickened or involved with fluorescein leakage, the number of lipid exudates, whether cysts are present on fluorescein angiography, and thickness of the central subfield on OCT.

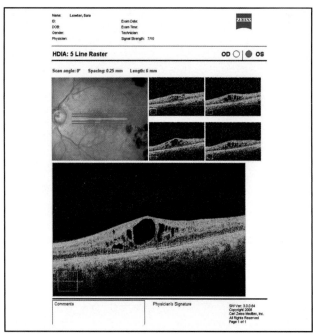

Figure 7-9. OCT showing fluid-filled cysts splitting the perifoveal neuroretina.

The list of published definitions for focal and diffuse diabetic macular edema is large, and the potential confusion arising from so many possible meanings for the 2 terms is apparent. The Global Diabetic Retinopathy Project Group based its definition of diabetic macular edema on clinical examination results alone, without reference to the terms *focal* or *diffuse*. This group defined diabetic macular edema as "present" or "absent" based on thickening or lipid exudates in the macula. When present, diabetic macular edema was subclassified into mild, moderate, or severe, depending on the distance of the thickening and exudates from the fovea.[13] Little evidence exists that characteristics of diabetic macular edema described by the terms *focal* and *diffuse* help explain variation in visual acuity or response to treatment. It is unresolved whether a concept of focal and diffuse diabetic macular edema will prove clinically useful despite frequent use of the terms when describing management of diabetic macular edema.

A working group within the Diabetic Retinopathy Clinical Research Network (DRCR.net) has been attempting to clarify the terms *focal* and *diffuse* diabetic macular edema. Its purpose is to determine whether definitions can be developed that are clinically applicable and reproducible. Until more rigorous studies have been carried out to investigate the issues discussed, authors writing about diabetic macular edema should use the terms *focal* and *diffuse* with caution, providing clear definitions that can be replicated by others.

Pathophysiology of Diabetic Macular Edema

In the physiologic state, water is produced as a metabolic byproduct within the neuronal tissue. Metabolic activity produces water as the end product of electron removal and adenosine triphosphate (ATP) generation.[14] The normal intraocular pressure of the eye continuously forces fluid into the retina. The force generated by this fluid entering the retina is one of the mechanisms that maintains the attachment of the retina to the retinal pigment epithelium (RPE).[15]

Under normal conditions, the inner retina is continuously dehydrated by glial cells, such as Müller cells, whereas the subretinal space and outer retina are kept dry by the pumping mechanism of the RPE. For the purpose of the movement of water through retinal tissue and RPE, these cells are endowed with special water channels known as aquaporins,[16] which enhance the permeability of membranes and mediate rapid and extensive fluid exchange. Intraretinal fluid collection may develop as a result of enhanced fluid leakage due to breakdown of the blood-retinal barrier or by the impaired removal of fluid from the retinal tissue into the systemic circulation. This barrier is formed by the vascular endothelium of the retinal vessels and the tight junctions between RPE cells. A breakdown of this barrier results in fluid accumulation within the retina and subretinal space. Generally, the edema may develop due to fluid collection in interstitial spaces (extracellular fluid) causing cellular compression, or it may collect within cells (intracellular), resulting in cellular swelling. Once excess fluid has entered the retinal interstitium, its further spread is limited by 2 high-resistant barriers against fluid movement, the inner and outer plexiform layers.[17] The layers may act as barriers as the extracellular space within them is highly convoluted and very narrow, thereby preventing free passage of fluid and solutes.

A prevailing view is that cyst formation secondary to macular edema is formed by swollen and dying Müller cells. In intracellular edema, leakage will not be seen on angiography, as the fluid is intracellular. An explanation of intracellular edema in diabetes is provided by the hypoxia-induced K+ channel disturbances. The redistribution of K+ channels results in a net accumulation of K+ ions within cells, building an osmotic gradient. This gradient drives water from the blood and vitreous into the glial cells via aquaporins and causes glial swelling, edema, and cyst formation.[18,19]

When present as cysts, the fluid-filled cysts are predominantly located in the inner nuclear layer and Henle fiber layer. This fluid accumulation results in cell displacement and the splitting of the perifoveal neuroretina within these layers (see Figure 7-9). On OCT and histology, Müller cell fibers are seen spanning these fluid-filled compartments.[20]

STRUCTURAL RETINAL CHANGES

Thickening of Capillary Basement Membrane

The basement membrane of the microvasculature thickens in diabetes mellitus. This change has been duplicated in numerous animal models of the disease.[21] The sorbitol pathway has been implicated as a cause for this thickening.[22] This change is not specific to the microvasculature of the retina although its prevention by the use of aldol reductase (AR) inhibitors is specific to retinal tissue in animal models. The exact influence of this structural change on the formation of macular edema is still unknown and under current research.

Loss of Microvascular Pericytes

The highest density of pericytes in the body is seen in the vasculature of the central nervous system and retina.[23] The microvasculature pericyte was first described in 1873; however, it is a cell that has largely been ignored in the clinical literature by its more famous neighbor, the endothelial cell. It has long been held that pericytes are particularly susceptible to the insults of diabetes and are lost more rapidly than endothelial cells. Pericytes are multifunctional, polymorphic, perivascular cells that lie within and contribute to the production of the microvessel basil lamina, and are the second cells that comprise the capillary wall in a prime location to be involved with microvascular permeability. They are capable of regulating blood flow in capillary beds, as they can produce vasoconstriction and vasodilation in these blood vessels. Changes in pericyte contractility alter the physical capillary barrier by opening the endothelial junctional space.[24] Pericytes have receptors for and respond to adrenergic and cholinergic stimulation, and they regulate permeability through contractility and apoptosis. Pericyte (and endothelial) cell death by apoptosis leads to a compromise of the barrier effect of the capillary wall.

The exact sequence of events in macular edema is not thoroughly understood, although pericyte loss contributes to increased permeability and is the primary physiological abnormality seen in the early stages. This "pericyte dropout" causes the vascular walls to weaken and generate microaneurysms, which in turn become a source of leakage into the retina.

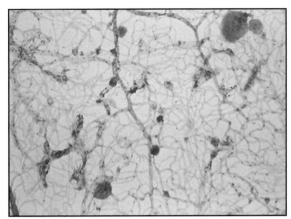

Figure 7-10. Retinal microaneurysms are one of the earliest clinical changes and most characteristic ophthalmoscopic features that are recognized in diabetic retinopathy.

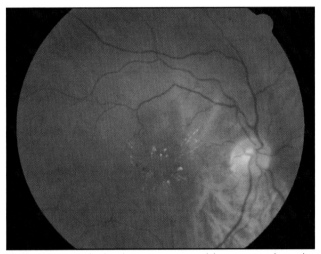

Figure 7-11. Retinal microaneurysms arising temporal to the macula.

Microaneurysm

Retinal microaneurysms are one of the earliest clinical changes and the most characteristic ophthalmoscopic feature that can be recognized in diabetic retinopathy (Figure 7-10). Although they occur in a number of systemic disorders, they do so more frequently in diabetic retinopathy. They can arise anywhere throughout the posterior pole, but often are first noted temporal to the macula, where blood vessels are present mostly in the inner nuclear layer of the retina (Figure 7-11). Their importance lies in their association with retinopathy severity and as sources for leakage of fluid and lipid transudates. Histologically, they are outpouchings of the capillaries with focal endothelial cell proliferation and pericyte loss, often adjacent to areas of no perfusion (Figure 7-12).[24] These areas of nonperfusion weaken the vessel wall and allow the pressure of the intravascular blood to form an outpouching, which is seen as a microaneurysm. The focal proliferation of endothelial

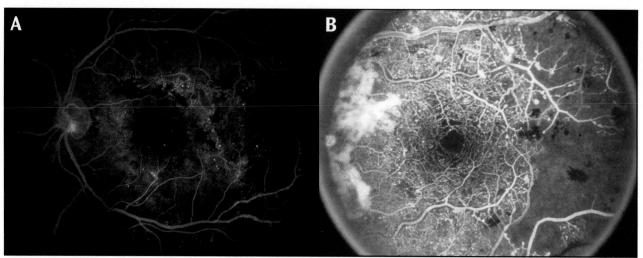

Figure 7-12. Retinal microaneurysms adjacent to areas of retinal nonperfusion.

cells secondary to the loss of antiproliferative effects of pericytes has also been cited as a reason for their formation,[25,26] in addition to other factors such as loss of supporting astrocytes, hemodynamic alterations (increased capillary intramural pressure), and local production of vasoproliferative factors such as vascular endothelial growth factor (VEGF).

The Blood–Retinal Barrier

The retina is insulated from the systemic circulation by the existence of the blood-retinal barrier. This barrier has an inner and outer component: the inner at the vascular endothelium of the intrinsic retinal circulation and the outer at the RPE. Another component of the inner barrier is the lack of intraendothelial vesicles in the retinal vasculature. In the macula, the retinal vessels are surrounded by the Müller glial cells that control the barrier properties of the endothelial cells. Two major types of proteins that form an important part of this barrier are occludins and claudins. Other proteins that serve a barrier function belong to the zonula occludens group. Experimental removal or alteration of these proteins results in an increase in permeability of small molecules across these barriers.[27] Three cellular mechanisms lead to blood-retinal barrier breakdown: leakage through the tight junctions of retinal vascular endothelium or RPE, upregulation of vesicular transport, and permeation of the surface membranes (fenestrations) of the cells that constitute the blood-retinal barrier. Multiple growth factors, such as hepatocyte growth factor, fibroblast growth factor, and insulin-like growth factor (IGF), and cytokines, such as histamine, tumor necrosis factor (TNF), interleukin (IL) B, and VEGF, contribute to vascular permeability by disrupting the tight junction proteins in the endothelium.

Experts agree that diabetic retinopathy originates with hyperglycemia. Abundant evidence demonstrates that elevated glucose levels in the retina initiate a complex series of responses, some independent and some interrelated, that ultimately lead to the characteristic microvascular changes seen in the diabetic retina. Several major lines of research have attempted to elucidate the connection between hyperglycemia and microvascular damage. These include increased polyol pathway flux, advanced glycation end products (AGEs), activation of protein kinase C (PKC), increased hexosamine pathway flux, and activation of the renin-angiotensin system. The unified theory of diabetic retinopathy postulates that many of these pathways ultimately lead to increased oxidative stress due to the formation of reactive oxygen species (ROS). Increasingly, evidence highlights the contribution of neurodegeneration and inflammation, as well as angiogenesis, in the pathogenesis of diabetic retinopathy.

The Polyol Pathway

Activation of the polyol pathway occurs when glucose levels rise in the bloodstream, as happens among patients with diabetes. When glucose levels are high, the enzyme AR reduces glucose to an osmotically active polyol alcohol, sorbitol. Nicotinamide adenine dinucleotide phosphate (NADPH) functions as a cofactor in this process. As NADPH is consumed processing glucose to sorbitol, it therefore becomes less available to regenerate reduced glutathione. NADPH eventually reconstitutes as sorbitol and ultimately converts to fructose; however, its reduced availability to regenerate glutathione has been postulated as a contributor to oxidative stress.[22]

Advanced Glycation End Products

AGEs develop under hyperglycemic conditions. They are generated from early glycation end products and are the final product of the nonenzymatic reaction of proteins and reducing sugars. They are generated from early glycation end products that result from altered glucose metabolism. Elevated levels of AGEs interfere with multiple processes within the retina. An increase in AGEs in diabetic blood vessels alters extracellular matrix components and integrins and disrupts matrix-cell interactions. AGEs also decrease the number of healthy pericytes and promote capillary permeability and blood-retinal barrier breakdown. Researchers note an increase in receptor-mediated production of ROS associated with elevated levels of AGEs.[28,29]

The Renin–Angiotensin System

A functioning renin-angiotensin system is located in the retinal circulation of the human eye. Renin is synthesized in RPE and retinal Müller cells. The renin-angiotensin system affects vascular smooth muscle cells and the accumulation of extracellular matrix proteins. It affects diabetic retinopathy at the local ocular level and systemic level, influencing blood pressure in the body. The activated renin-angiotensin system in diabetes has received extensive attention as an important pathway in microvascular damage. In fact, pharmacologic inhibition of the renin-angiotensin system can delay onset of early retinopathy, reduces intracellular uptake of glucose, and improves retinal blood flow abnormalities; however, it has little effect on progression of retinopathy in the more advanced stages.[30]

Protein Kinase C

Hyperglycemia indirectly activates many of the 11 isoforms of diacylglycerol (DAG) PKC throughout retinal tissues. An elevation of DAG is seen in diabetes. DAG in turn activates the enzyme, PKC. The β-isoform of PKC (PKC-β) mediates the effects of elevated DAG. The complex cascade of reactions to elevated PKC involves alterations in cellular signaling via modifications in signal transduction and increases in VEGF. Vascular changes include perturbations in blood flow, leukocyte vascular adhesion, and vascular permeability. Increased extracellular matrix protein expansion results from synthesis of type IV collagen, TGF-β1, and fibronectin.[30-32]

Other Possible Mechanisms of Diabetic Macular Edema

Increased flux through the hexosamine pathway occurs when intracellular glucose levels are high. Activation of this pathway results in altered gene activation and modifications in gene transcription that are associated with vascular endothelial dysfunction.

Inflammatory mediators including proinflammatory cytokines and chemokines lead to chronic, low-grade inflammation in the diabetic retina. Leukocytes drawn to the retina accumulate, and elevated levels of factors such as TNF-α increase leukocyte-endothelial cell adhesion. The resultant leukostasis worsens capillary nonperfusion and endothelial cell damage.

Several investigations have demonstrated upregulation of cyclooxygenase-2 (COX-2) in tissues affected by diabetes; these findings may help delineate the mechanisms underlying chronic inflammation and microvascular damage in diabetes.

ANCILLARY DIAGNOSTIC TESTS

Color fundus photography, fluorescein angiography, OCT, and ultrasonography, in addition to the clinical examination, are important in the evaluation and management of diabetic retinopathy. Diabetic macular edema is a diagnosis made clinically during the ophthalmic retinal evaluation. Ancillary tests are used only to confirm, guide, and/or follow up its treatment. However, these diagnostic studies are useful for adequate documentation and as a guide to the appropriate treatment and follow-up.

Color Stereo Fundus Photographs

Color fundus photography is an important tool that can be used to document retinal findings in patients with diabetes (Figure 7-13).[33] It can be used for tracking the progression of the disease and also in some instances for the screening of diabetic retinopathy.[34] Several studies have compared a variety of examining and imaging techniques with 7-field stereoscopic fundus photographs. Among these, the most common is comparing dilated fundus examinations and fundus photographs to detect the presence and severity of diabetic retinopathy.[35] Generally, the photographic protocol has been found to be more sensitive than either direct or indirect ophthalmoscopy, but similar to slit-lamp biomicroscopy carried out by an experienced and highly motivated examiner.[36]

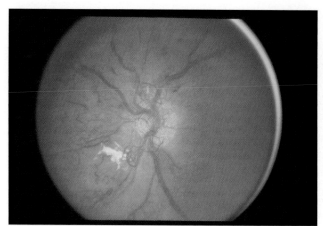

Figure 7-13. Color fundus photograph of a patient with diabetes showing areas of microaneurysms, neovascularization of the disc, and lipid exudates.

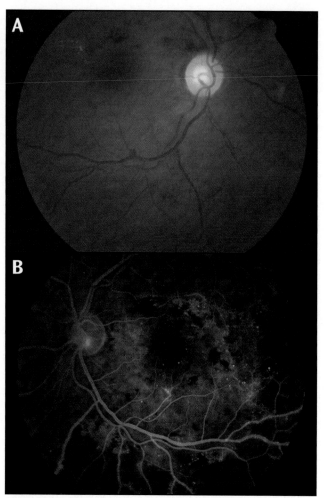

Figure 7-14. Photographs of the retinal periphery showing areas of neovascularization in a patient with diabetes.

For comparison purposes, it is essential that photographs be produced in a consistent, standardized manner (ie, similar exposure and field of view). Color fundus photography may be obtained in either a stereoscopic or nonstereoscopic fashion, depending on the capabilities of the camera. Fundus photography can be performed in the traditional 7 stereoscopic 30-degree fields or wide-angle 60-degree fields. Both 30- and 60-degree fields have advantages and disadvantages, but in general, the 7 stereoscopic 30-degree fields provide the most complete coverage, and the 60-degree view is useful in more advanced proliferative disease with vitreous traction. In some instances, fundus photography can be used at the initial examination and may be repeated either to document significant progression of disease or track responses to treatment (Figure 7-14).

The use of color photography as a screening option for diabetic retinopathy has been studied and implemented.[37,38] The significance of detecting clinically important lesions of retinopathy is to facilitate the timely administration of treatment strategies to prevent vision loss. In patients with CSME, the challenge is to detect the elevation of the retinal fovea by photographic means. This would require either viewing or photographing the affected eye using stereoscopic methods. Both CSME and PDR may require dilated eye examinations to obtain adequate ophthalmoscopy or quality photographs to assess for the presence of these fine vessels.

A growing number of studies have been conducted with digital photography, as clinical practice has converted to digital for many ophthalmologists. The ease of performance as well as the ease in storage makes digital photography more desirable. The gold standard for the documentation of diabetic retinopathy consists of stereoscopic photography of 7 standard fields on color film established in the ETDRS.[6]

The desire of the ophthalmology community to capture wide-field images of the fundus is long-standing.[39,40] The evaluation of many retinal diseases including diabetes depends partly, and at times entirely, on imaging the peripheral fundus. The width of the composite setting obtained from multiple 30-degree retinal images is approximately 75 degrees (Figure 7-15). Photographs anterior to the equator may be obtained, but such photography is limited by patient alignment problems, focus irregularities, marginal corneal astigmatism, poor fixation, and light reflex artifacts. Newer noncontact camera systems may capture images up to 50 degrees across; however, peripheral images still must be manually pasted together by the practitioner to formulate a composite.

In 1992, a novel ellipsoidal mirror with dual focal points, one of which lies posterior to the iris plane, was developed (Optos P200 MA, Optos plc, Dunfermline, UK). The combination of this mirror with a noncontact scanning laser ophthalmoscope (non-cSLO) imaging platform now allows rapid acquisition of 200-degree

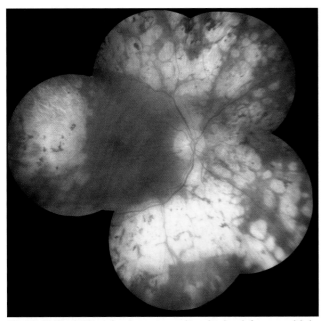

Figure 7-15. Retinal fundus composite obtained from multiple 30-degree retinal images at a width of 75 degrees.

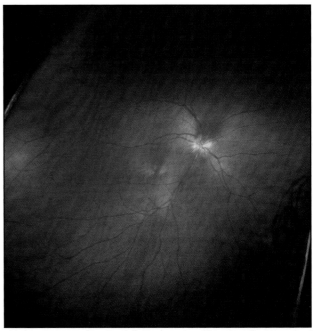

Figure 7-16. Two hundred-degree panoramic color photograph of the retinal fundus.

panoramic retinal fundus images (Figures 7-16 and 7-17). Retinal microvascular injury in diabetes results in pericyte loss, endothelial cell apoptosis, capillary hyperpermeability, and capillary nonperfusion, which eventually manifest findings such as diabetic macular edema, retinal ischemia, and neovascularization. It has long been established that diabetic ischemia and capillary nonperfusion occur commonly in the midperiphery,[41] which is why the use of wide angle retinal photography becomes an important diagnostic tool when treating these patients because the identification of specific areas of nonperfused retina (Figures 7-18 and 7-19) may allow targeted rather than pan photocoagulation in the treatment of neovascularization. If more laser is required, it can be applied in a step-wise logical manner, therefore preserving more healthy retinal tissue, avoiding additional complications from the laser treatment itself, and enhancing the control of diabetic macular disease as well.

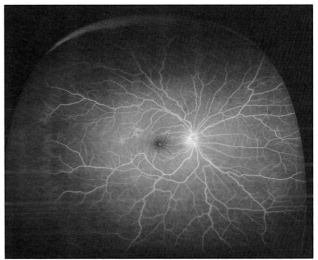

Figure 7-17. Two hundred-degree panoramic photograph of a fluorescein angiography.

Fluorescein Angiography

Novotny and Alvis[42] developed the present technique of fluorescein angiography. Although orally administered fluorescein has been attempted, intravenous administration is still the exclusive standard for acceptable resolution. Sodium fluorescein, which is protein-bound to albumin, is the dye used in fluorescein angiography. It diffuses freely through the choriocapillaries, Bruch membrane, optic nerve, and sclera. However, it does not diffuse through the tight junctions of the retinal endothelial cells, RPE, and larger choroidal vessels. A physiologic inner blood-retinal barrier exists at the retinal capillaries due to the tight junctions (zonula occludens) within these vessels. If the inner blood-retinal barrier is disrupted, dye leakage occurs. The tight junctions between the RPE cells constitute the outer blood-retinal barrier, which under normal nonpathologic conditions, is also impermeable to fluorescein.

Fluorescein angiographic quality depends on technique, filters, film, ocular media, and patient cooperation. Lenticular opacities, such as cataracts, scatter light, and the yellow lens absorbs the blue excitation

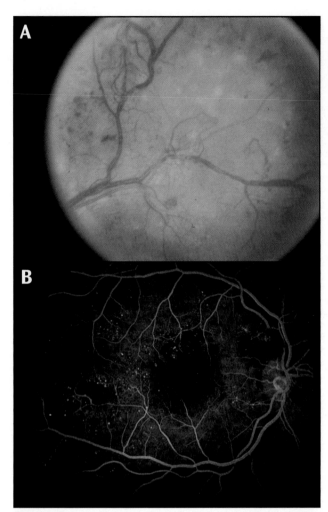

Figure 7-18. Area of retinal nonperfusion with neovascularization elsewhere.

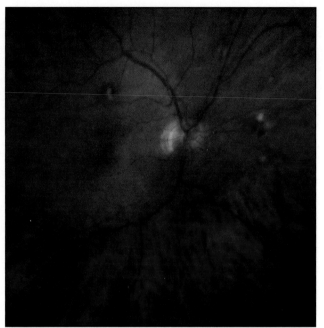

Figure 7-19. Diabetic macular edema in the presence of peripheral retinal ischemia.

light. Media opacities, such as vitreous hemorrhage, also impair the fluorescein test. By contrast, a remarkably normal study can be obtained through asteroid hyalosis. The most important uses of fluorescein angiography in diabetic retinopathy are guiding treatment of CSME and evaluating unexplained visual loss.[43]

Fluorescein angiography does not have a role in the screening of patients with diabetic retinopathy but could be occasionally used to determine the extent of peripheral capillary nonperfusion and search for subtle areas of neovascularization.[43]

Although sodium fluorescein is generally safe, severe anaphylactic reactions can occur in some patients at a rate of 1 in 200,000.[44]

Optical Coherence Tomography

To date, time domain OCT using the Stratus OCT has been the most widely used technique for obtaining macular measurements[45] and has been shown in previous studies to generate measurements with high repeatability.[46] This instrument acquires images of the vitreoretinal interface, retina, and subretinal space at a rate of 400 axial scans per second, with an axial resolution of 10 μm (Figure 7-20).

A new class of OCT devices using spectral (Fourier) domain technology has been developed. Although both time domain Stratus and spectral domain OCT use the same basic principles, the scan rate of spectral domain OCT is at least 20,000 axial scans per second, with improved axial resolution of 5 μm (Figure 7-21).

Forooghian et al demonstrated that the spectral domain OCT provided significantly higher macular thickness and volume measurements than the Stratus OCT.[47] The 2 OCT devices cannot be used interchangeably for the measurement of macular thickness and volume. The higher image resolution afforded by spectral domain OCT over Stratus OCT may show the former to be superior in the visualization of macular structure; the similar reliability of these systems makes them comparable in measuring the thickness and volume of the macula with statistical analysis.[47]

Lammer et al also compared different spectral domain OCT devices regarding retinal thickening values in eyes with diabetic macular edema and correlated the results with conventional time domain stratus OCT data.[48] They found that although interdevice reproducibility was satisfactory, retinal thickness and volume measurements should not be used interchangeably because measurements differed significantly between systems. The lack of interdevice agreement seems to be related to the different segmentation algorithm of thickness measurement and should be considered because it may strongly influence treatment decisions and conclusions.[48]

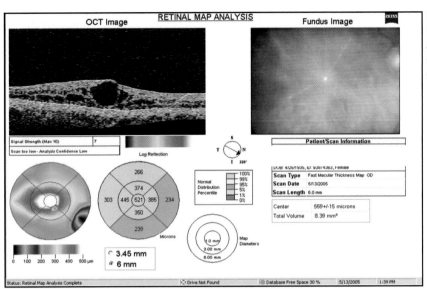

Figure 7-20. Stratus OCT (Carl Zeiss Meditec) images of the vitreoretinal interface, retina, and subretinal space at a rate of 400 axial scans per second, with an axial resolution of 10 μm.

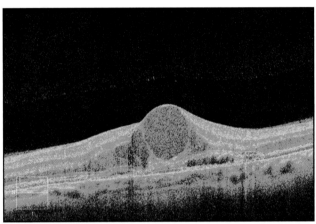

Figure 7-21. Although both time domain and spectral domain OCT use the same basic principles, the scan rate of spectral domain OCT is at least 20,000 axial scans per second, with improved axial resolution to 5 μm.

OCT can be useful for quantifying retinal thickness, monitoring macular edema, and identifying vitreomacular traction in selected patients with diabetic macular edema. However, OCT measures of retinal thickness correlate poorly with visual acuity.[49,50] Although it has long been appreciated that central macular thickness can be associated with a decrease in visual acuity and treatments that reduce such retinal thickening can improve vision, quantitative evaluation of these relationships and the effect of laser photocoagulation are scarce.

Browning et al documented substantial variation in visual acuities at any given retinal thickness.[49] Many eyes with a macula of normal thickness had decreased visual acuity. Their results suggested that OCT measurement alone may not be a good surrogate for visual acuity as a primary outcome in studies of diabetic macular edema. They concluded that assessment of macular thickness using OCT is clinically useful, but macular thickness is just one of several variables affecting visual acuity in a complex and as yet not fully understood relationship.

The DRCR.net evaluated OCT measurements and methods of analysis of OCT data in studies of diabetic macular edema.[51] This study concluded that central subfield, defined as the circular area of diameter 1 mm centered around the center point (128 thickness measurements in the fast mac protocol), was the preferred OCT measurement for the central macula because of its higher reproducibility and correlation with other measurements of the central macula. Total macular volume may be preferred when the central macula is less important. Absolute change in retinal thickness, defined as the difference in the thickness between 2 measurements made at different times, is the preferred analysis method in studies involving eyes with mild macular thickening. Relative change in retinal thickening, defined as the absolute change in thickness (or thickening) divided by the baseline thickening, may be preferable when retinal thickening is more severe.[51]

TREATMENT OPTIONS FOR DIABETIC MACULAR EDEMA

Systemic Control

The severity of hyperglycemia is the key modifiable risk factor associated with the development of diabetic retinopathy. Support of this association is found in results of both clinical trials and epidemiology studies.[52] Duration of diabetes and severity of hyperglycemia are the major risk factors for developing retinopathy. Once retinopathy is present, duration of diabetes appears to be a less important factor than hyperglycemia for progression from earlier to later stages of retinopathy.[53] Intensive management of hypertension has been demonstrated to slow retinopathy progression.[54] Elevated serum lipid levels are associated with the development of retinopathy.[55]

A 2010 study from the ACCORD Eye Study Group investigated whether intensive glycemic control, combination therapy for dyslipidemia, and intensive blood pressure control would limit the progression of diabetic retinopathy in persons with type 2 diabetes.[56] This study enrolled 10,251 participants with type 2 diabetes who were at high risk for cardiovascular disease to receive either intensive or standard treatment for glycemia (target glycated hemoglobin level, <6.0% or 7.0% to 7.9%, respectively) and also for dyslipidemia (160 mg daily of fenofibrate plus simvastatin or placebo plus simvastatin) or for systolic blood pressure control (target, <120 or <140 mm Hg). A subgroup of 2856 participants was evaluated for the effects of these interventions at 4 years on the progression of diabetic retinopathy by 3 or more steps on the ETDRS severity scale, or the development of diabetic retinopathy necessitating laser photocoagulation or vitrectomy.

At 4 years, the rates of progression of diabetic retinopathy were 7.3% with intensive glycemia treatment versus 10.4% with standard therapy (adjusted odds ratio [OR], 0.67; 95% confidence interval [CI], 0.51 to 0.87; P=.003); 6.5% with fenofibrate for intensive dyslipidemia therapy versus 10.2% with placebo (adjusted OR, 0.60; 95% CI, 0.42 to 0.87; P=.006); and 10.4% with intensive blood pressure therapy versus 8.8% with standard therapy (adjusted OR, 1.23; 95% CI, 0.84 to 1.79; P=.29).

The study concluded that intensive glycemic control and intensive combination treatment of dyslipidemia, but not intensive blood pressure control, reduced the rate of progression of diabetic retinopathy.[56]

Less agreement exists among studies concerning the importance of other factors such as age, type of diabetes, clotting factors, renal disease, physical inactivity, and use of angiotensin-converting enzyme inhibitors.[57-60] Many of these factors are associated with the substantial cardiovascular morbidity and mortality and other complications associated with diabetes. Thus, it is reasonable to encourage patients with diabetes to be as compliant as possible with therapy of all medical aspects of their disease.[61]

Retinal Laser Photocoagulation

Clinically significant macular edema is defined by the ETDRS to include any of the following features[5-8]:

- Thickening of the retina at or within 500 μm of the center of the macula, which is approximately one-half the optic disc diameter.

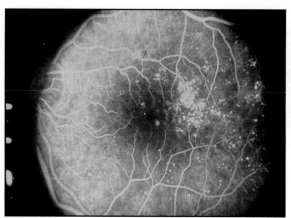

Figure 7-22. Fluorescein angiography identifying treatable lesions.

- Hard exudates at or within 500 μm of the center of the macula, if associated with thickening of the adjacent retina (not residual hard exudates remaining after the disappearance of retinal thickening).

- A zone or zones of retinal thickening 1 disc area or larger, any part of which is within 1 disc diameter of the center of the macula.

It is convenient to subdivide CSME according to involvement at the center of the macula because the risk of visual loss and the need for focal photocoagulation is greater when the center is involved. The diagnosis of diabetic macular edema can be difficult. Macular edema is best evaluated by dilated examination using slit-lamp biomicroscopy, OCT, and/or stereoscopic fundus photography. An ophthalmologist who treats patients for this condition should be familiar with relevant studies and techniques as described in the ETDRS.

- Fluorescein angiography prior to laser surgery for CSME often is helpful in identifying treatable lesions (although it is less important when circinate lipid exudates are present, in which leaking lesions often are obvious within the lipid ring) and pathologic enlargement of the foveal avascular zone, which may be useful in planning treatment (Figure 7-22).

- Color fundus photography is often helpful to document the status of the retina even if surgery is not performed (see Ancillary Diagnostic Tests section; Figure 7-23).

- OCT is helpful to detect subtle edema and follow the course of edema after treatment but is not necessary as a screening tool (Figure 7-24).

Patients with CSME should be considered for laser surgery. The risk of moderate visual loss is reduced by >50% for patients who undergo appropriate laser photocoagulation surgery compared with those who are not treated (Figures 7-25 and 7-26; Table 7-1).

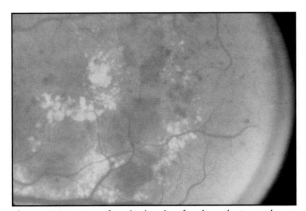

Figure 7-23. Use of retinal color fundus photography as an important tool documenting retinal findings in patients with diabetes. (Figure 7-26 illustrates areas of retinal thickening, hemorrhage, and lipid exudates close to the center of the macula in a patient with diabetes.) (Reprinted with permission of Flynn HR Jr, Smiddy WE. *Diabetes and Ocular Disease: Past, Present, and Future Therapies (Ophthalmology Monographs #14)*. San Francisco, CA: The Foundation of the American Academy of Ophthalmology; 2000:241.)

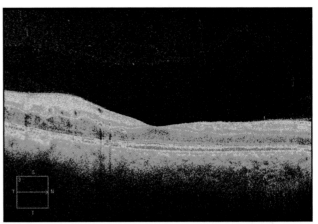

Figure 7-24. OCT showing subtle edema after focal laser treatment.

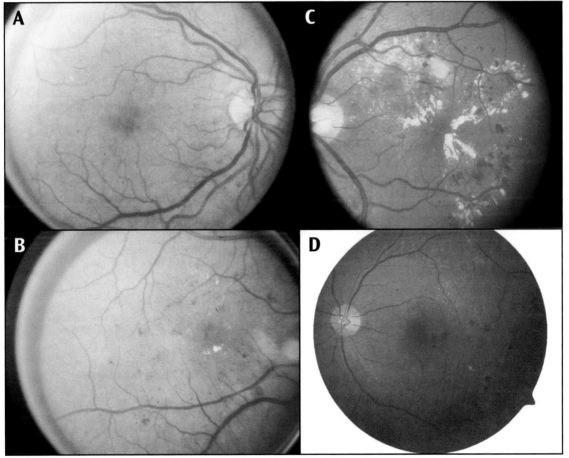

Figure 7-25. Color fundus photographs documenting clinically significant diabetic macular edema prior to treatment with argon laser photocoagulation.

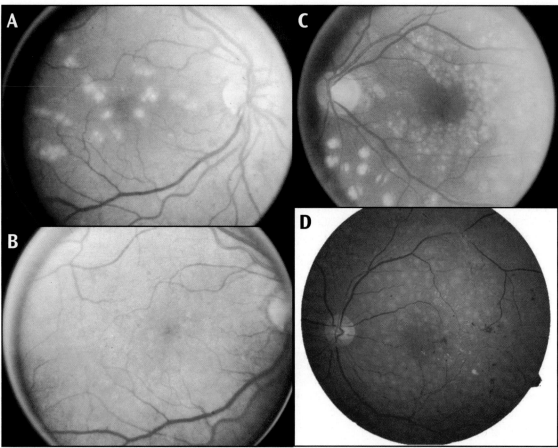

Figure 7-26. Color fundus photographs documenting resolved diabetic macular edema after treatment with argon laser photocoagulation.

Table 7-1. Early Treatment Diabetic Retinopathy Study[5-8,43]

1. Study Questions

1.1 Is photocoagulation effective for treating diabetic macular edema?
1.2 Is photocoagulation effective for treating diabetic retinopathy?
1.3 Is aspirin effective for preventing progression of diabetic retinopathy?

2. Eligibility

2.1 Mild nonproliferative diabetic retinopathy through early proliferative diabetic retinopathy, with visual acuity 20/200 or better in each eye.

3. Randomization

3.1 3711 participants: 1 eye randomly assigned to photocoagulation (scatter and/or focal) and 1 eye assigned to no photocoagulation; patients randomly assigned to 650 mg/d aspirin or placebo.

4. Outcome Variables

4.1 Visual acuity worse than 5/200 for at least 4 months; visual acuity worsening by doubling the initial visual angle (eg, 20/40 to 20/80); retinopathy progression.

5. Aspirin Use Results

5.1 Aspirin use did not alter progression of diabetic retinopathy.
5.2 Aspirin use did not increase risk of vitreous hemorrhage.
5.3 Aspirin use did not affect visual acuity.
5.4 Aspirin use reduced risk of cardiovascular morbidity and mortality.

6. Early Scatter Photocoagulation Results

6.1 Early scatter photocoagulation resulted in small reduction in risk of severe visual loss (worse than 5/200 for at least 4 months)
6.2 Early scatter photocoagulation is not indicated for eyes with mild to moderate diabetic retinopathy.
6.3 Early scatter photocoagulation may be most effective in patients with type 2 diabetes.

7. Macular Edema Results

7.1 Focal photocoagulation for diabetic macular edema decreased risk of moderate visual loss (doubling of initial visual angle).
7.2 Focal photocoagulation for diabetic macular edema increased chance of moderate visual gain (halving of initial visual angle).
7.3 Focal photocoagulation for diabetic macular edema reduced retinal thickening.

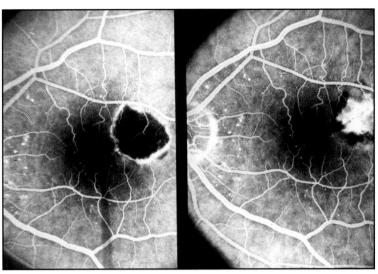

Figure 7-27. Juxtafoveal laser scar extending into the fovea as a complication of prior focal laser photocoagulation.

Vision improves for a minority of patients. For the majority of cases, the goal of treatment with laser photocoagulation is to stabilize the visual acuity. Patients with CSME and excellent visual function should be considered for treatment before visual loss occurs.

Analyses of the ETDRS data showed that following laser photocoagulation, improvement in vision occurred in patients with initial visual acuity worse than 20/40, whereas those with initial vision better than 20/40 had less room to show an improvement. Most patients require more than one treatment session (3 to 4 on average), 2 to 4 months apart, for macular edema to resolve. When treatment is deferred, as may be desirable when the center of the macula is not involved or imminently threatened, the patient should be observed closely (at least every 3 to 4 months) for progression.

Rarely, focal laser photocoagulation may induce subretinal fibrosis with choroidal neovascularization, which may be associated with permanent central vision loss. The most important factors associated with subretinal fibrosis include the most severe degree of subretinal hard exudates in the macula and elevated serum lipids prior to laser photocoagulation. Only 8% of cases of subretinal fibrosis were directly related to focal laser photocoagulation.[62]

Effective laser treatment and retreatment protocols have been detailed in the Diabetic Retinopathy Study (DRS) and the ETDRS.[5-8,63] Preoperatively, the ophthalmologist should discuss the side effects and treatment risks with the patient. A follow-up examination for individuals with CSME should be scheduled within 2 to 4 months of laser surgery.

Several types of wavelengths with different characteristics can be used for macular laser treatment. The green wavelength (argon, DF-Nd:YAG) is better absorbed by the hemoglobin. The red/infrared wavelength (krypton, diode) produces less damage to the inner retina and is better focused if the media is opaque. Theoretically, longer wavelengths of photocoagulation have the added advantage that transmission through the human cornea and lens are significantly higher in the red and infrared region compared with the blue end.[64] This advantage reduces problems of attenuation of radiation by pre-target absorption or scatter. Infrared irradiation reduces the intraocular scatter or "blue light scatter."[65] The negligible absorption of near infrared radiation within the yellow xanthophyll pigment of the macula provides an additional protective advantage over irradiation with shorter wavelengths in the visible portion of the spectrum. However, in clinical studies, no evidence exists regarding any difference among the efficacies of the different wavelengths.[66]

The most frequent complications of traditional retinal laser therapy are paracentral scotomas, accidental foveal photocoagulation, juxtafoveal laser scars that enlarge into the fovea, choroidal neovascularization, and subfoveal fibrosis. Atrophy of the RPE can result in expansion of the laser scar to a spot 200% larger than the intended original spot size (Figure 7-27).[66] This enlarged area of atrophy can result in loss of central vision, central scotoma, and decreased color vision. Therefore, it is advisable to use lighter, less intense laser burns than originally specified by the ETDRS.[67]

Macular laser alone has been shown to compromise quality of vision by affecting contrast sensitivity, color vision, or central visual field.[68] Another risk of focal or grid laser is the development of choroidal neovascularization (Figure 7-28). This risk is related to the rupture of Bruch membrane from the laser spot and could be decreased by choosing a bigger spot size or by using less energy and longer duration of laser delivery.[69]

The development of the micropulsed diode laser has allowed the production of subthreshold, clinically invisible scars in the treatment of diabetic macular edema.[70] The diode laser emits in the near infrared spectrum

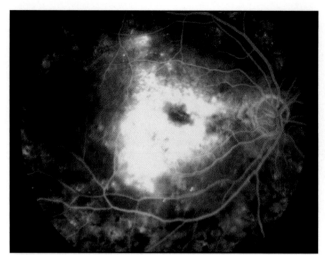

Figure 7-28. Choroidal neovascularization with subfoveal fibrosis as a complication of prior focal laser photocoagulation.

and, similar to other retinal lasers, is absorbed by the RPE. The relative absorption of diode laser light at 800 nm in the RPE is approximately 40% of that of argon at 488 nm.[71] Clinical studies showed that this was sufficient to produce therapeutic effects.[71,72] The comparable clinical effects with argon laser confirm the fact that the underlying concept of laser photocoagulation is derived from processes dependent on energy deposition in the RPE and not due to focal deposition of thermal energy at sites of vascular leakage. Diode laser has poor absorption within hemoglobin and thus a limited direct effect on vascular leakage.[72]

The morphological advantages of the subthreshold diode laser are the absence of visible scars. Functional advantages include the absence of scotomas, preservation of color vision, and contrast sensitivity. The limitation of the procedure is the difficulty in titrating the end point, given that no ophthalmoscopically visible way exists to confirm the effect of the treatment. Follow-up of patients who have undergone laser treatment is every 3 to 4 months. The retreatment decision is based on the persistence of thickening, as seen by biomicroscopy, and leakage recorded by fluorescein angiography. OCT is helpful in quantifying retinal thickness changes and identifying vitreoretinal traction.[73]

Animal models of diabetic retinopathy demonstrate that inflammation plays an important role.[73] In early onset of diabetic retinopathy, upregulation of COX-2 occurs in retinal cells. This results in elevated prostaglandin production, leading to an increased expression of VEGF and an increased risk of vascular leakage and retinal neovascularization.[74] High-dose aspirin and intermediate doses of COX-2 inhibitors (celecoxib) were apparently beneficial in early experimental diabetic retinopathy. Based on these past experiences, Chew et al[75] designed a prospective, randomized, multicenter trial comparing COX-2 inhibitor (celecoxib) with

placebo and diode grid laser with standard ETDRS focal laser treatment in 86 patients with diabetic macular edema. The micropulse diode technique was conducted with the 810 diode laser (Iris Medical OcuLight SLx; IRIDEX Corp, Mountain View, CA) by using the MicroPulse operating mode. The treatment consisted of 125-µm-sized burns using a 10% duty cycle with 0.2-s pulse envelope duration with a maximum power of 1.8 W. These were subthreshold burns that covered the entire area of macular edema with minimal clinical detection of fluorescein angiography changes associated with these laser burns. The primary outcome included a 50% reduction in the retinal thickening of diabetic macular edema measured with OCT (Stratus OCT) and a 50% reduction of leakage severity determined on fluorescein angiography.

This study was prematurely terminated because of safety concerns of celecoxib treatment, reported by the National Institutes of Health, for all participants in a large colorectal cancer prevention clinical trial in which a 2- to 3-fold increased risk of major fatal and nonfatal cardiovascular events was found for participants taking celecoxib compared with those in the placebo group.[76] This early termination also reduced the power of the study because the projected sample size of 100 was not achieved, with only 86 participants.

Visual acuity and retinal thickening data collected over 2 years of follow-up did not show differences between the medical and laser treatments. However, participants assigned to the celecoxib group were more likely to have a reduction in fluorescein angiography leakage compared with the placebo group (P<.01). The overall conclusion was that no significant visual function benefits of treatment with celecoxib or diode laser were noted compared with those of standard laser treatment, but a suggestive effect of celecoxib in reducing fluorescein angiography leakage was observed.[75]

Micropulse and subthreshold photocoagulation have been reported to produce equally effective or improved visual outcomes compared to standard modified ETDRS laser treatment.[76,77] However, the absence of visible laser uptake may prompt inappropriate higher power laser titration or unnecessary retreatment. A new system named Pascal (pattern scanning laser) Photocoagulator (Optimedica Corp, Santa Barbara, CA) is a semi-automated laser delivery system that reduces procedural time by delivering multiple laser burns with a single application.[78] Importantly, medium pulse duration (10 to 20 ms) may result in less destruction to the outer retina, compared with conventional laser burns, presumably because of reduced axial and lateral thermal spread.[79]

Despite recent knowledge of the Pascal therapeutic parameters, benchmark laser parameters for treating diabetic macular edema have yet to be demonstrated in randomized clinical trials. Muqit et al published data on the use of Pascal photocoagulation burns in diabetic macular edema determined by Fourier-domain OCT and fundus autofluorescence.[80] Their study concluded that barely visible, 10-ms Pascal laser seems to produce an effect at the level of the inner and outer photoreceptor segments and apical RPE, with minimal axial and lateral spread of burns. Fourier-domain OCT confirmed spatial localization of autofluorescence signal changes that correlated with laser burn-tissue interactions over 3 months. The technique of lower fluence, barely visible, 10-ms Pascal macular laser photocoagulation may produce highly localized retinal lesions and effective treatment outcomes for patients with diabetic macular edema. Fourier-domain OCT in combination with autofluorescence may be useful 1 hour after laser treatment to confirm laser burn application, while showing the extent of the treated area. Autofluorescence thereafter may be used as a monitoring tool for barely visible treatments, either to confirm successful placement of burns or to plan retreatments for recurrent, persistent diabetic macular edema. Barely visible, 10-ms Pascal macular laser photocoagulation may induce less tissue damage than conventional threshold laser photocoagulation while retaining therapeutic properties.[80]

Several recent and ongoing studies compared the efficacy of laser with other treatments such as intravitreal injection of various medications such as steroids and anti-VEGF drugs as well as combination therapies to determine whether any additional benefits are present in terms of efficacy and interval of treatments. (These studies are discussed in the section on Intravitreal Injection Pharmacotherapy).

Pars Plana Vitrectomy

Multiple case series have indicated that pars plana vitrectomy to manage selected patients with diffuse CSME that is unresponsive to previous macular laser photocoagulation may improve visual acuity when substantial vitreomacular traction is present. However, the value of vitrectomy in CSME has not been studied in a randomized clinical trial.[81,82]

A 2010 publication, by the DRCRN Writing Committee on behalf of the DRCR.net, evaluated vitrectomy for diabetic macular edema in eyes with at least moderate vision loss and vitreomacular traction.[83] The prospective cohort study included 87 eyes with diabetic macular edema and vitreomacular traction based on investigators' evaluation, visual acuity 20/63 to 20/400, OCT central subfield >300 μm, and no concomitant cataract extraction at the time of vitrectomy. These investigators concluded that after vitrectomy performed for diabetic macular edema and vitreomacular traction, retinal thickening was reduced in most eyes. Between 28% and 49% of eyes with characteristics

similar to those included in the study are likely to have improvement of visual acuity, whereas between 13% and 31% are likely to have worsening. The operative complication rate is low and similar to what has been reported for this procedure. Their data provided estimates of surgical outcomes and serve as a reference for future studies that might consider vitrectomy for diabetic macular edema in eyes with at least moderate vision loss and vitreomacular traction.

Intravitreal Injection Pharmacotherapy

Role of Corticosteroids

Proliferative diabetic retinopathy and diabetic macular edema are the primary causes of visual loss in diabetic patients.[84,85] Panretinal photocoagulation (PRP) as treatment for PDR was first introduced more than 40 years ago.[86] The safety and effectiveness of PRP has been validated by many studies, including the DRS (Table 7-2) and ETDRS (see Table 7-1).[87,88] PRP is the only established treatment modality for PDR proven to consistently induce long-term quiescence and prevent further visual loss in patients with PDR.[89]

In contrast, standard treatment for diabetic macular edema is somewhat less effective and more variable in outcome.[90] Diabetic macular edema can be present at any stage of diabetic retinopathy and is the leading cause of moderate visual loss, afflicting nearly 1.2 million individuals in the United States alone.[91] The use of focal laser photocoagulation as the standard of care for treatment of diabetic macular edema was established more than 20 years ago by the findings of the ETDRS and remains the standard to which novel treatments are compared.[5-8]

The broad biologic activity and multiple pharmacologic effects of corticosteroids supported the rationale behind their use for treatment of diabetic macular edema. Corticosteroids have been found to inhibit both VEGF and VEGF gene expression.[92] Their anti-inflammatory activity in part relies on blocking the release of arachidonic acid from cell membrane and reducing the synthesis of inflammatory prostaglandins.[93] They have also been shown to inhibit migration of leukocytes and stabilize the endothelial cell tight junctions.[94] Based on these studies, various investigators successfully used steroids (triamcinolone acetonide), off label, to treat diabetic macular edema through intravitreal injections.[95,96] The initial case series and small, uncontrolled, randomized, clinical trials observed a rapid and often dramatic reduction in macular thickness and improvement in visual acuity.[97-100] The effect was transient and required repeated injections, which were associated with an increased rate of steroid-related complications such as cataract progression and elevated intraocular pressure.

Table 7-2. Diabetic Retinopathy Study (1972-1979)[63,87,88]

Visual Outcome for Xenon Arc and Argon Laser Photocoagulation From the Diabetic Retinopathy Study

Baseline Severity of Retinopathy	Duration of Follow-up (y)	Control Patients (% With Severe Visual Loss)	Treated Patients (% With Severe Visual Loss)
Severe NPDR	2	3	3
	4	13	4
Mild PDR	2	7	3
	4	21	7
High-risk PDR	2	26	11
	4	44	20

The Diabetic Retinopathy Study (DRS) was designed to investigate the value of xenon and argon laser photocoagulation for patients with severe nonproliferative diabetic retinopathy (NPDR) and proliferative diabetic retinopathy (PDR).

A small, prospective, 6-month clinical trial published in 2006[101] used a single 4-mg intravitreal injection for diffuse diabetic macular edema unresponsive to focal/grid laser treatment. Treatment with 4-mg intravitreal injection reduced macular thickness at 1 month (intravitreal injection 228 μm, no injection 501 μm; P<.001) and 3 months (intravitreal injection 211 μm, no injection 444 μm; P<.001). However, no difference was observed in macular thickness at 6 months in eyes with intravitreal injection compared to eyes that were not injected (358 and 441 μm, respectively; P>0.1). Intravitreal injected eyes were observed to have gained more ETDRS letters at 1, 3, and 6 months, but at 7 months, the visual benefit from intravitreal injection was no longer significant (P=.17). All study eyes had previously received and were unresponsive to focal/grid laser treatment prior to participation in the study. The study did not use a laser control arm; consequently, the benefit observed cannot be directly compared to laser.

Gillies at al[100] were the first to report 2-year results of a double-masked, placebo-controlled, randomized, clinical trial of 4-mg intravitreal injection in eyes with diabetic macular edema and impaired vision that persisted or recurred after laser treatment. Over the study period, it was shown that intravitreal injection treatment substantially reduced the need for further laser treatment (P=.0001), with a mean improvement of 5.7 ETDRS letters, and an overall shift toward greater visual gain in eyes treated with intravitreal injection compared to placebo. Furthermore, foveal thickness in eyes treated with intravitreal injection decreased 59 μm more than eyes treated with placebo. This study clearly showed that in eyes with center-involved diabetic macular edema unresponsive to focal laser treatment, intravitreal injection treatment improved vision and reduced

macular thickness over a 2-year period compared to no treatment. Once again, no laser control arm was included in this study. An improvement of >5 letters in 26% of placebo and 56% of eyes treated with intravitreal injection led the authors to conclude that spontaneous improvement, similar to that observed with the original ETDRS control arm, could still occur in eyes that have been severely affected by diabetic macular edema.[100]

The potential clinical importance of corticosteroids in the treatment of diabetic macular edema was recognized by the National Eye Institute-supported DRCR.net, which conducted 2 steroid-related, prospective, randomized, clinical trials. The initial DRCR.net trial evaluated both anterior and posterior subtenon injections of triamcinolone acetonide and did not show any benefit for the treatment of diabetic macular edema in eyes with either normal or slightly reduced visual acuity.[102] An earlier, smaller randomized trial in patients having worse visual acuity compared to the population in the DRCR.net trial showed equivocal results.[103] Due to these findings, pursuit of a larger phase III trial of peribulbar or subtenon steroids for diabetic macular edema was abandoned.[102]

The second DRCR.net trial evaluated the efficacy and safety of intravitreal injection compared to focal/grid photocoagulation using a prospective, multicenter, randomized design. A meta-analysis of earlier randomized controlled trials had shown intravitreal injection to have a significant short-term benefit in the treatment of diabetic macular edema.[97] The DRCR.net conducted a 2-year, multicenter, randomized, controlled study of intraocular preservative-free triamcinolone acetonide. At 4 months, it was observed that eyes treated with 1- and 4-mg intravitreal injection had greater improvement in corrected visual acuity when compared to focal/grid photocoagulation.[82] However, by 1 year, no significant differences in corrected visual acuity were noted among the 3 groups. Beginning at 16 months and extending to the primary outcome at 2 years, the laser group had a greater improvement in corrected visual acuity than the intravitreal injection groups.

The effect on macular thickness was generally similar to that of visual acuity. The 4-mg intravitreal injection group achieved an initial rapid dramatic reduction in macular thickness at 4 months compared to laser and 1-mg intravitreal injection. At 2 years, as observed in the visual acuity findings, the trend reversed and the laser group had a greater reduction in macular thickness compared to both intravitreal injection groups. The larger reduction in macular thickness in the laser group was present regardless of the degree of retinal thickness at baseline.[82]

The visual outcome in all 3 treatment groups appeared to be better than the untreated natural course, although this was not evaluated specifically in this study. However, a nearly 4-fold increase in the rate of intraocular pressure elevation and need for cataract surgery was observed in the steroid treatment groups.[82]

Adjunctive use of triamcinolone acetonide in the treatment of diabetic macular edema has received considerable attention. Lam et al evaluated the efficacy of sequential intravitreal injection followed by grid laser for treating diabetic macular edema.[104] Patients were randomized to grid laser, 4 mg of intravitreal injection, or 4 mg of intravitreal injection combined with sequential grid laser after 1 month. The authors concluded that combined treatment may enhance the short-term efficacy of laser by inducing a greater reduction in macular thickness, but recurrence of diabetic macular edema is common and a greater reduction in macular thickness does not necessarily translate into improved vision.[104]

Avitabile et al performed a similar prospective, 3-arm, randomized, clinical trial comparing efficacies of intravitreal injection, grid laser alone, and sequential intravitreal injection followed by grid laser 3 months later.[105] Patients were observed for a mean of 9 months, and it was demonstrated that eyes treated with 4-mg intravitreal injection with or without additional grid laser had significantly larger reduction in macular edema and better mean final visual acuity than eyes treated with laser alone.[105] No significant differences in macular thickness and visual acuity were found between the intravitreal injection-alone group and eyes treated with combined intravitreal injection and laser at all time points. This led authors to conclude that additional laser photocoagulation after intravitreal injection might not provide an additional benefit.[105]

Kang et al compared the outcomes of intravitreal injection combined with grid laser after 3 weeks to intravitreal injection without laser in patients with diffuse diabetic macular edema. Patients who received grid laser after intravitreal injection were found to have significantly better corrected visual acuity and a greater reduction in macular thickness at 3 and 6 months after treatment. The authors concluded that combined grid laser and intravitreal injection maintains improved visual acuity and reduces the recurrence of diabetic macular edema.[106]

A 3-year follow-up report by the DRCR.net[107] of a randomized trial comparing focal/grid photocoagulation laser treatment and intravitreal injection for diabetic macular edema was consistent with previously published 2-year results[82] and did not indicate a long-term benefit of intravitreal injection relative to focal/grid photocoagulation in patients with diabetic macular edema. Rather, visual acuity outcomes slightly favored the laser group over the 2 triamcinolone groups. The investigators indicated that most eyes receiving 4 mg of intravitreal injection are likely to require cataract surgery, although only a few will develop glaucoma requiring surgery.[107]

The treatment of PDR with PRP remains the current standard of care, being the only modality proven to effectively reduce the long-term incidence of visual loss.[89] When PDR occurs concurrently with CSME, management becomes more complex. PRP can cause or worsen CSME,[6] but the extent to which this happens under current treatment regimens is unknown and is being evaluated in ongoing studies.[108] The stabilization of diabetic retinal neovascularization with corticosteroid treatment alone has not yet been reported. Small prospective trials have shown potentially promising results with the addition of intravitreal injection to PRP in the management of PDR and CSME.[109]

Role of Vascular Endothelial Growth Factor Inhibitors

VEGF has been identified as one of the many growth factors causing breakdown on the blood-retinal barrier with increased retinal permeability by affecting the endothelial tight junctions.[110] Although normal human retina contains VEGF, the levels are significantly elevated in eyes with diabetic macular edema, with hypoxia and hyperglycemia as contributing factors.[74,111] As a result, pharmacologic attenuation of the effects of VEGF using several anti-VEGF therapies such as pegaptanib (Macugen) and ranibizumab (Lucentis) have been hypothesized and anecdotally tested as alternative treatments, and all have shown favorable short-term results.[112,113]

Bevacizumab (Avastin), a humanized monoclonal antibody that neutralizes all VEGF isoforms, was originally approved by the US Food and Drug Administration (FDA) for the treatment of metastatic colorectal cancer in 2004.[114] The off-label use of intraretinal bevacizumab has been applied to many diseases in the eye, particularly age-related macular degeneration, PDR, neovascular glaucoma, diabetic macular edema, retinopathy of prematurity, and macular edema secondary to retinal vein occlusions.[115,116] Although not currently approved by the FDA for intravitreal use, the injection of 1.25 to 2.5 mg of intravitreal bevacizumab has been performed without significant intraocular toxicity.[117]

Goyal et al, in an attempt to gain a better perspective on a systematic review highlighting the evidence for the therapeutic effect and safety of bevacizumab in the treatment of diabetic macular edema, performed a meta-analysis and review of randomized clinical trials performed prior to July 2009 to quantify the effect of bevacizumab on visual acuity and central macular thickness in diabetic macular edema, as well as the adverse events described with this therapy.[118] Their meta-analysis substantiated the short-term beneficial effects of intravitreal bevacizumab compared to standard laser therapy.[118] Intravitreal bevacizumab caused significant reduction in central subfield macular thickness (CSMT) and improvement in visual acuity at 6 weeks compared to macular photocoagulation. However, no statistically meaningful difference was noted in CSMT or visual acuity between the study and control groups at 12 weeks. At 24 weeks, the combined results from 2 trials showed a significant improvement in vision without a significant decrease in CSMT. Furthermore, their analysis suggested no significant benefit of adding steroids to bevacizumab for improving either the anatomical (CSMT) or functional (visual acuity) aspect of diabetic macular edema at any time. The use of intravitreal injection should be considered carefully because of cumulative side effects such as cataract and glaucoma and the potential toxicity of the drug itself.[118]

The emerging popularity of anti-VEGF agents is also raising concerns about safety with long-term use of these agents. Because bevacizumab is a full-length immunoglobulin, it remains in the systemic circulation significantly longer than ranibizumab, raising the possibility of both local and systemic overdosage, particularly with an already compromised blood-retinal barrier.[119] Bevacizumab, as a pan-VEGF blocker, has the potential to inhibit important physiological functions of VEGF such as wound healing and development of collaterals deemed significant in myocardial or peripheral ischemia, thus potentially causing systemic adverse events.[120]

The DRCR.net published a randomized, multicenter, clinical study evaluating intravitreal injection of 0.5 mg ranibizumab and 4 mg triamcinolone combined with focal/grid laser compared with focal/grid laser alone for the treatment of diabetic macular edema.[121] Eyes were randomized to placebo injection plus prompt laser, 0.5 mg ranibizumab plus laser, 0.5 mg ranibizumab plus deferred laser, or 4 mg triamcinolone plus prompt laser. The main outcome measured was corrected visual acuity and safety at 1 year. Their results showed that intravitreal injection of ranibizumab with prompt or deferred laser was more effective through at least 1 year compared with prompt laser alone for the treatment of diabetic macular edema involving the central macula, resulting in superior visual acuity and OCT outcomes compared with focal/grid laser treatment without ranibizumab.[121]

Overall, intravitreal triamcinolone combined with focal/grid laser did not result in superior visual acuity outcomes compared with laser without triamcinolone, although it resulted in a greater reduction in retinal thickening at 1 year but not at 2 years compared with laser alone. However, in an analysis limited to pseudophakic eyes, the triamcinolone plus prompt laser group outcome for visual acuity was of similar magnitude to that of the 2 ranibizumab groups, suggesting that cataract formation, cataract surgery, or both may have affected visual acuity outcomes adversely among phakic eyes in the triamcinolone plus prompt laser group.[121]

If ranibizumab is to be given as it was applied in the study by the DRCR.net, the 1- and 2-year data show a need to follow eyes continuously undergoing this treatment because the results indicate that additional ranibizumab, focal/grid laser, or both are needed in most eyes through at least 2 years, even if "success" criteria are met early in the course of treatment. The authors did not find any evidence that ranibizumab or triamcinolone were associated with an increased risk of systemic side effects or overall mortality, including cerebrovascular and cardiovascular events. However, in view of the low number of observed events, a small increased risk cannot be ruled out.[121]

Other studies are underway that are comparing intravitreal ranibizumab alone or in combination with laser, with laser alone over 1 year,[122] and intravitreal ranibizumab alone with placebo injection.[123,124] Results from these and other studies should complement knowledge regarding the safety and efficacy of ranibizumab and other anti-VEGF drugs, alone or in combination with laser, for the treatment of diabetic macular edema.

In conclusion, focal/grid laser has been the mainstay of treatment for diabetic macular edema during the past 25 years. On the basis of the data from the DRCR. net protocol, intravitreal ranibizumab with deferred (24 weeks) or prompt focal/grid laser is superior to focal/grid laser alone for the treatment of diabetic macular edema involving the center of the macula through at least 1 year of follow-up, with significantly more eyes gaining substantial vision and significantly fewer eyes losing substantial vision.[117] In pseudophakic eyes, intravitreal triamcinolone with prompt focal/grid laser may be equally effective as ranibizumab at improving visual acuity and reducing retinal thickening but is associated with an increased risk of elevated intraocular pressure. Further follow-up is needed to determine long-term safety and efficacy of ranibizumab in the treatment of diabetic macular edema.

SUMMARY

The clinically optimal treatment of diabetic macular edema has not yet been realized. Focal/grid laser treatment remains the primary treatment option in the management of center-involved diabetic macular edema. Future efforts to optimally address the treatment of diabetic macular edema must recognize that the pathogenesis of diabetic macular edema may be multifactorial, involving such diverse processes as inflammation, angio/vasculogenesis, junctional mechanisms, and actions of a variety of different and possibly independent growth/permeability factors. Combination therapies, targeting multiple distinct pathophysiologic pathways may eventually prove necessary for maximal efficacy. In addition, because the relative contributions of these specific mechanisms may vary among individuals or possibly over time in the same individual, ultimately treatment regimens may need to be tailored to the unique disease profile of the individual patient.

ACKNOWLEDGMENTS

I would like to acknowledge Dr. Arnaldo Espaillat, medical director of the Instituto Espaillat Cabral, and Dr. Rosina Negrin, Chief of the Retina Department at the same institution, in Santo Domingo, Dominican Republic, for providing many of the images published in this chapter.

REFERENCES

1. Browning DJ. *Diabetic Retinopathy Evidence-Based Management*. New York, NY: Springer; 2010.
2. Williams R, Airey M, Baxter H, Forrester J, Kennedy-Martin T, Girach A. Epidemiology of diabetic retinopathy and macular oedema: a systemic review. *Eye*. 2004;18:963-983.
3. Wild S, Roglic G, Green A, Sicree R, King H. Global prevalence of diabetes: estimates for the year 2000 and projections for 2030. *Diabetes Care*. 2004;27:1047-1053.
4. Klein R, Klein BE, Moss SE, Cruickshanks KJ. The Wisconsin Epidemiologic Study of Diabetic Retinopathy: XVII. The 14-year incidence and progression of diabetic retinopathhy. associated risk factors in type 1 diabetes. *Ophthalmology*. 1998;105:1801-1815.
5. Chew EY, Klein MI, Murphy RP, Remaley NA, Ferris FL III. Effects of aspirin on vitreous/preretinal hemorrhage in patients with diabetes mellitus. Early Treatment Diabetic Retinopathy Study report no 20. *Arch Ophthalmol*. 1995;113:52-55.
6. Early Treatment Diabetic Retinopathy Study Research Group. Early photocoagulation for diabetic retinopathy. ETDRS Report 9. *Ophthalmology*. 1991;98:766-785.
7. Ferris F. Early photocoagulation in patients with either type I or type II diabetes. ETDRS Report 24. Early Treatment Diabetic Retinopathy Study Research Group. *Trans Am Ophthalmol Soc*. 1996;94:505-537.
8. Flynn HW Jr, Chew EY, Simons BD, Barton FB, Remaley NA, Ferris FL III. Pars plana vitrectomy in the Early Treatment Diabetic Retinopathy Study. ETDRS Report 17. Early Treatment Diabetic Retinopathy Study Research Group. *Ophthalmology*. 1992;99:1351-1357.
9. Browning DJ, Altaweel MM, Bressler NM, Bressler SB, Scott IU. Diabetic macular edema: what is focal and what is diffuse? *Am J Ophthalmol*. 2008;146:649-655.
10. Laursen ML, Moeller F, Sander B, Sjoelie AK. Subthreshold micropulse diode laser treatment in diabetic macular edema. *Br J Ophthalmol*. 2004;88:1173-1179.
11. Catier A, Tadayoni R, Paques M, et al. Characterization of macular edema from various etiologies by optical coherent tomography. *Am J Ophthalmol*. 2005;140:200-206.
12. Jensen DB, Knudsen LL. Stereoscopic fluorescein angiography in diabetic maculopathy. *Retina*. 2006;26:153-158.
13. Wilkinson CP, Ferris FL III, Klein RE, et al. Proposed international clinical diabetic retinopathy and diabetic macular edema disease severity scale. *Ophthalmology*. 2003;110:1677-1682.
14. Murray RK, Granner DK, Mayes PA, et al. The respiratory chain and oxidative phosphorylation. In: Foltin J, Ransom J, Oransky JM, eds. *Harper's Illustrated Biochemistry*. 26th ed. New York, NY: McGraw-Hill Companies; 2003:92-101.
15. Fatt I, Shantinath K. Flow conductivity of retina and its role in retinal adhesion. *Exp Eye Res*. 1971;12:218-226.
16. Nagelhus EA, Veruki ML, Torp R, et al. Aquaporin-4 channel protein in the rat retina and optic nerve: polarized expression in Muller cells and fibrous astrocytes. *J Neurosci*. 1998;18:2506-2519.
17. Antcliff RJ, Hussain AA, Marshall J. Hydraulic conductivity of fixed retinal tissue after sequential excimer laser ablation: barriers limiting fluid distribution and implications for cystoids macular edema. *Arch Ophthalmol*. 2001;119:539-544.
18. Bringmann A, Reichenbach A, Wiedemann P. Pathomechanisms of cystoid macular edema. *Ophthalmic Res*. 2004;36:241-249.
19. Pannicke T, Iandiev I, Uckermann O, et al. A potassium channel-linked mechanism of glial cell swelling in the postischemic retina. *Mol Cell Neurosci*. 2004;26:493-502.
20. Antcliff RJ, Marshall J. The pathogenesis of edema in diabetic retinopathy. *Semin Ophthalmol*. 1999;14:223-232.
21. Hainsworth DP, Katz ML, Sanders DA, Sanders DN, Wright EJ, Sturek M. Retinal capillary basement membrane thickening in a porcine model of diabetes mellitus. *Comp Med*. 2002;52:523-529.
22. Takamura Y, Tomomatsu T, Kubo E, Tsuzuki S, Akagi Y. Role of the polyol pathway in high glucose induced apoptosis of retinal pericytes and proliferation of endothelial cells. *Invest Ophthalmol Vis Sci*. 2008;49:3216-3223.
23. Edelman DA, Jiang Y, Tyburski J, Wilson RF, Steffes C. Pericytes and their role in microvascular homeostasis. *J Surg Res*. 2006;135:305-11.
24. Moore J, Bagley S, Ireland G, McLeod D, Boulton ME. Three dimensional analysis of microaneurysms in the human diabetic retina. *J Anat*. 1999;194:89-100.
25. Orlidge A, D'Amore PA. Inhibition of capillary endothelial cell growth by pericytes and smooth muscle cells. *J Cell Biol*. 1987;105:1455-1462.
26. Lindahl P, Johansson BR, Levéen P, Betsholtz C. Pericyte loss and microaneurysm formation in PDGF-B-deficient mice. *Science*. 1997;277:242-245.

27. Antonetti DA, Barber AJ, Khin S, Lieth E, Tarbell JM, Gardner TW. Vascular permeability in experimental diabetics is associated with reduced endothelial occluding content: vascular endothelial growth factor decreases occluding in retinal endothelial cells. Penn State Retina Research Group. *Diabetes*. 1998;47:1953-1959.

28. Stii AW, Li YM, Gardiner TA, Bucala R, Archer DB, Vlassara H. Advanced glycation end products (AGEs) colocalize with AGE receptors in the retinal vasculature of diabetic and of AGE-infused rats. *Am J Pathol*. 1997;150:523-531.

29. Barile GR, Pachydaki SI, Tari SR, et al. The RAGE axis in early diabetic retinopathy. *Invest Ophthalmol Vis Sci*. 2005; 46:2916-2924.

30. Perkins BA, Aiello LP, Krolewski AS. Diabetes complications and the renin–angiotensin system. *N Engl J Med*. 2009;361:83-85.

31. Koya D, King GL. Protein kinase C activation and the development of diabetic complications. *Diabetes*. 1998;47:859-866.

32. Aiello LP, Bursell SE, Clermont A, et al. Vascular endothelial growth factor-induced retinal permeability is mediated by protein kinase C in vivo and suppressed by an orally effective β-isoform-selective inhibitor. *Diabetes*. 1997;46:1473-1480.

33. Klein R, Klein BE, Neider MW, Hubbard LD, Meuer SM, Brothers RJ. Diabetic retinopathy as detected using ophthalmoscopy, a nonmydriatic camera and a standard fundus camera. *Ophthalmology*. 1985;92:485-491.

34. Moss SE, Klein R, Kessler SD, Richie KA. Comparison between ophthalmoscopy and fundus photography in determining severity of diabetic retinopathy. *Ophthalmology*. 1985; 92:62-67.

35. Emanuele N, Klein R, Moritz T, et al. Comparison of dilated fundus examinations with seven-field stereo fundus photographs in the Veterans Affairs Diabetes Trial. *J Diabetes Complications*. 2009;23:323-329.

36. Scanlon PH, Malhotra R, Greenwood RH, et al. Comparison of two reference standards in validating two field mydriatic digital photography as a method of screening for diabetic retinopathy. *Br J Ophthalmol*. 2003;87:1258-1263.

37. Chow SP, Aiello LM, Cavallerano JD, et al. Comparison of nonmydriatic retinal imaging versus dilated ophthalmic examination for nondiabetic eye disease in persons with diabetes. *Ophthalmology*. 2006;113:833-840.

38. Chew EY. Screening options for diabetic retinopathy. *Curr Opin Ophthalmol*. 2006;17:519-522.

39. Lotmar W. A fixation lamp for panoramic fundus pictures. *Klin Monatsbl Augenheilkd*. 1977;170:767-774.

40. Noyori KS, Chino K, Deguchi T. Wide field fluorescein angiography by use of contact lens. *Retina*. 1983;3:131-134.

41. Kimble JA, Brandt BM, McGwin G Jr. Clinical examination accurately locates capillary nonperfusion in diabetic retinopathy. *Am J Ophthalmol*. 2005;139:555-557.

42. Novotny HR, Alvis DL. A method of photographing fluorescein in the human retina. *Circulation*. 1961;24:72-77.

43. Diabetic Retinopathy. *Preferred Practice Pattern*. San Francisco, CA: American Academy of Ophthalmology; 2008.

44. Yannuzzi LA, Rohrer KT, Tindel LJ, et al. Fluorescein angiography complication survey. *Ophthalmology*. 1986;93:611-617.

45. Jaffe GJ, Caprioli J. Optical coherent tomography to detect and manage retinal disease and glaucoma. *Am J Ophthalmol*. 2004;137:156-169.

46. Massin P, Vicaut E, Haouchine B, Erginay A, Paques M, Gaudric A. Reproducibility of retinal mapping using optical coherence tomography. *Arch Ophthalmol*. 2001;119:1135-1142.

47. Forooghian F, Cukras C, Meyerle CB, Chew EY, Wong WT. Evaluation of time domain and spectral domain optical coherent tomography in the measurement of diabetic macular edema. *Invest Ophthalmol Vis Sci*. 2008;49:4290-4296.

48. Lammer J, Scholda C, Prünte C, Benesch T, Schmidt-Erfurth U, Bolz M. Retinal thickness and volume measurements in diabetic macular edema: a comparison of four optical coherent tomography systems. *Retina*. 2011;31:48-55.

49. Browning DJ, Glassman AR, Aiello LP, et al. Relationship between optical coherence tomography-measured central retinal thickness and visual acuity in diabetic macular edema. *Ophthalmology*. 2007;114:525-536.

50. Virgili G, Menchini F, Dimastrogiovanni AF, et al. Optical coherence tomography versus stereoscopic fundus photography or biomicroscopy for diagnosing diabetic macular edema: a systematic review. *Invest Ophthalmol Vis Sci*. 2007;48:4963-73.

51. Browning DJ, Glassman AR, Aiello LP, et al. Optical coherence tomography measurements and analysis methods in optical coherence tomography studies of diabetic macular edema. *Ophthalmology*. 2008;115:1366-1371.

52. Diabetes Control and Complications Trial Research Group. Progression of retinopathy with intensive versus conventional treatment in the Diabetes Control and Complications Trial. *Ophthalmology*. 1995;102:647-661.

53. Davis MD, Fisher MR, Gangnon RE, et al. Risk factors for high-risk proliferative diabetic retinopathy and severe visual loss: Early Treatment Diabetic Retinopathy Study report number 18. *Invest Ophthalmol Vis Sci*. 1998; 39:233-252.

54. Snow V, Weiss KB, Mottur-Pilson C; Clinical Efficacy Assessment Subcommittee of the American College of Physicians. The evidence base for tight blood pressure control in the management of type 2 diabetes mellitus. *Ann Intern Med*. 2003;138:587-592.

55. Van Leiden HA, Dekker JM, Moll AC, et al. Blood pressure, lipids, and obesity are associated with retinopathy: the Hoorn Study. *Diabetes Care*. 2002;25:1320-1325.

56. ACCORD Study Group. Effects of medical therapies on retinopathy progression in type 2 diabetes. *N Engl J Med*. 2010;363:233-244.

57. Klein R, Klein BE, Moss SE, et al. The Wisconsin Epidemiologic Study of Diabetic Retinopathy. IX. Four-year incidence and progression of diabetic retinopathy when age at diagnosis is less than 30 years. *Arch Ophthalmol*. 1989;107:237-243.

58. Klein R, Klein BE, Moss SE, et al. The Wisconsin Epidemiologic Study of Diabetic Retinopathy. X. Four-year incidence and progression of diabetic retinopathy when age at diagnosis is 30 years or more. *Arch Ophthalmol*. 1989;107:244-249.

59. Kriska AM, LaPorte RE, Patrick SL, et al. The association of physical activity and diabetic complications in individuals with insulin-dependent diabetes mellitus: the Epidemiology of Diabetes Complications Study--VII. *J Clin Epidemiol*. 1991;44:1207-1214.

60. American Diabetes Association. Standards of medical care in diabetes--2008. *Diabetes Care*. 2008;31(Suppl 1):S12-S54.

61. The Diabetic Retinopathy Study Research Group. Indications for photocoagulation treatment of diabetic retinopathy: Diabetic Retinopathy Study report number 14. *Int Ophthalmol Clin*. 1987;27:239-253.

62. Brancato R, Pece A, Avanza P, Radrizzani E. Photocoagulation scar expansion after laser therapy for choroidal neovascularization in degenerative myopia. *Retina*. 1990;10(4):239-243.

63. The Diabetic Retinopathy Study Research Group. Four risk factors for severe visual loss in diabetic retinopathy. The third report from the Diabetic Retinopathy Study. *Arch Ophthalmol*. 1979;97:654-655.

64. Lerman S. An experimental and clinical evaluation of lens transparency and aging. *J Gerontol*. 1983;38:293-301.

65. Akduman L, Olk RJ. Diode laser (810 nm) versus argon green (514) modified grid photocoagulation for diffuse diabetic macular edema. *Ophthalmology*. 1997;104:1433-1441.

66. Schatz H, Madeira D, McDonald HR, Johnson RN. Progressive enlargement of laser scars following grid laser photocoagulation for diffuse diabetic macular edema. *Arch Ophthalmol.* 1991;109:1549-1551.

67. Ahmadi AM, Lim JI. Update on laser treatment of diabetic macular edema. *Int Ophthalmol Clin.* 2009;49:87-94.

68. Morgan CM, Schatz H. Atrophic creep of the retinal pigment epithelium after focal macular photocoagulation. *Ophthalmology.* 1989;96:96-103.

69. Varley MP, Frank E, Purnell EW. Subretinal neovascularization after focal argón laser for diabetic macular edema. *Ophthalmology.* 1988;95:567-573.

70. Ulbig MW, McHugh DA, Hamilton AM. Diode laser photocoagulation for diabetic macular oedema. *Br J Ophthalmol.* 1995;79:318-321.

71. McHugh JD, Marshall J, Ffytche TJ, Hamilton AM, Raven A, Keeler CR. Initial clinical experience using a diode laser in the treatment of retinal vascular disease. *Eye.* 1989;3(Pt 5):516-527.

72. Bailey CC, Sparrow JM, Grey RH, Cheng H. The National Diabetic Retinopathy Laser Treatment Audit. III. Clinical outcomes. *Eye.* 1999;13(Pt 2):151-159.

73. Johnson EI, Dunlop ME, Larkins RG. Increased vasodilatory prostaglandin production in the diabetic rat retinal vasculature. *Curr Eye Res.* 1999;18:79-82.

74. Aiello LP, Avery RL, Arrigg PG, et al. Vascular endothelial growth factor in ocular fluid of patients with diabetic retinopathy and other retinal disorders. *N Engl J Med.* 1994;331:1480-1487.

75. Chew EY, Kim J, Coleman HR, et al. Preliminary assessment of celecoxib and microdiode pulse laser treatment of diabetic macular edema. *Retina.* 2010;30:459-467.

76. Solomon SD, McMurray JJ, Pfeffer MA, et al. Cardiovascular risk associated with celecoxib in a clinical trial for colorectal adenoma prevention. *N Engl J Med.* 2005;352:1071-1080.

77. Luttrul JK, Musch DC, Mainster MA. Subthreshold diode micropulse photocoagulation for the treatment of clinically significant diabetic macular oedema. *Br J Ophthalmol.* 2005;89:74-80.

78. Blumenkranz MS, Yellachich D, Andersen DE, et al. New instrument: semiautomated patterned scanning laser for retinal photocoagulation. *Retina.* 2006;26:370-375.

79. Jain A, Blumenkranz MS, Paulus Y, et al. Effect of pulse duration on size and character of the lesion in retinal photocoagulation. *Arch Ophthalmol.* 2008; 126:78-85.

80. Muqit MM, Gray JC, Marcellino GR, et al. Barely visible 10-millisecond pascal laser photocoagulation for diabetic macular edema: observations of clinical effect and burn localization. *Am J Ophthalmol.* 2010;149:979-986.e2.

81. Yamamoto T, Hitani K, Tsukahara I, et al. Early postoperative retinal thickness changes and complications after vitrectomy for diabetic macular edema. *Am J Ophthalmol.* 2003;135:14-19.

82. Diabetic Retinopathy Clinical Research Network. A randomized trial comparing intravitreal triamcinolone acetonide and focal/grid photocoagulation for diabetic macular edema. *Ophthalmology.* 2008;115:1447-1459, 1449.e1-e10.

83. Diabetic Retinopathy Clinical Research Network. Vitrectomy outcomes in eyes with diabetic macular edema and vitreomacular traction. *Ophthalmology.* 2010;117:1087-1093.

84. Centers for Disease Control and Prevention. National diabetes fact sheet: general information and national estimates on diabetes in the United States, 2007. Atlanta, GA: Department of Health and Human Services, Centers for Disease Control and Prevention; 2008.

85. Klein R, Klein BE. Vision disorders. In Harris MW, Ed. *Diabetes in America.* Bethesda, MD: NIH-NIDDK Publication No. 95-1468, 1995:293-338.

86. Beetham WP, Aiello LM, Balodimos MC, Koncz L. Ruby-laser photocoagulation of early diabetic neovascular retinopathy: preliminary report of a long-term controlled study. *Trans Am Ophthalmol Soc.* 1969;67:39-67.

87. The Diabetic Retinopathy Study Research Group. Photocoagulation treatment of proliferative diabetic retinopathy: the second report of Diabetic Retinopathy Study findings. *Ophthalmology.* 1978;85:82-106.

88. The Diabetic Retinopathy Vitrectomy Study Research Group. Early vitrectomy for severe vitreous hemorrhage in diabetic retinopathy. Two-year results of a randomized trial. Diabetic Retinopathy Vitrectomy Study report 2. *Arch Ophthalmol.* 1985;103:1644-1652.

89. Chew EY, Ferris FL III, Csaky KG, et al. The long-term effects of laser photocoagulation treatment in patients with diabetic retinopathy: the early treatment diabetic retinopathy study follow up study. *Ophthalmology.* 2003;110:1683-1689.

90. Silva PS, Sun JK, Aiello LP. Role of steroids in the management of diabetic macular edema and proliferative diabetic retinopathy. *Seminars in Ophthalmology.* 2009;24:93-99.

91. Klein R, Klein BE, Moss SE, et al. The Wisconsin epidemiologic study of diabetic retinopathy. IV. Diabetic macular edema. *Ophthalmology.* 1984;91:1464-1474.

92. Antonetti DA, Barber AJ, Hollinger LA, Wolpert EB, Gardner TW. Vascular endothelial growth factor induces rapid phosphorylation of tight junction proteins occluding and zonula occluden 1. A potential mechanism for vascular permeability in diabetic retinopathy and tumors. *J Biol Chem.* 1999;274:23463-23467.

93. Joussen AM, Smyth N, Niessen C. Pathophysiology of diabetic macular edema. *Dev Ophthalmol.* 2007;39:1-12.

94. Miyamoto K, Khosrof S, Bursell SE, et al. Prevention of leukostasis and vascular leakage in streptozotocin-induced diabetic retinopathy via intercellular adhesion molecule-1 inhibition. *Proc Natl Acad Sci USA.* 1999;96:10836-10841.

95. Jonas JB, Söfker A. Intraocular injection of crystalline cortisone as adjunctive treatment of diabetic macular edema. *Am J Ophthalmol.* 2001;132:425-427.

96. Martidis A, Duker JS, Greenberg PB, et al. Intravitreal triamcinolone for refractory diabetic macular edema. *Ophthalmology.* 2002;109:920-927.

97. Grover D, Li TJ, Chong CC. Intravitreal steroids for macular edema in diabetes. *Cochrane Database Syst Rev.* 2008;CD005656.

98. Ockrim ZK, Sivaprasad S, Falk S, et al. Intravitreal triamcinolone versus laser photocoagulation for persistent diabetic macular oedema. *Br J Ophthalmol.* 2008;92:795-799.

99. Massin P, Audren F, Haouchine B, et al. Intravitreal triamcinolone acetonide for diabetic diffuse macular edema: preliminary results of a prospective controlled trial. *Ophthalmology.* 2004;111:218-224.

100. Gillies MC, Sutter FK, Simpson JM, Larsson J, Ali H, Zhu M. Intravitreal triamcinolone for refractory diabetic macular edema: two-year results of a double-masked, placebo-controlled, randomized clinical trial. *Ophthalmology.* 2006;113:1533-1538.

101. Audren F, Erginay A, Haouchine B, et al. Intravitreal triamcinolone acetonide for diffuse diabetic macular oedema: 6-month results of a prospective controlled trial. *Acta Ophthalmol Scand.* 2006;84:624-630.

102. Diabetic Retinopathy Clinical Research Network, Chew E, Strauber S, et al. Randomized trial of peribulbar triamcinolone acetonide with and without focal photocoagulation for mild diabetic macular edema: a pilot study. *Ophthalmology.* 2007;114:1190-1196.

103. Entezari M, Ahmadieh H, Dehghan MH, Ramezani A, Bassirnia N, Anissian A. Posterior sub-tenon triamcinolone for refractory diabetic macular edema: a randomized clinical trial. *Eur J Ophthalmol*. 2005;15:746-750.

104. Lam DS, Chan CK, Mohamed S, et al. Intravitreal triamcinolone plus sequential grid laser versus triamcinolone or laser alone for treating diabetic macular edema: six-month outcomes. *Ophthalmology*. 2007;114:2162-2167.

105. Avitabile T, Longo A, Reibaldi A. Intravitreal triamcinolone compared with macular laser grid photocoagulation for the treatment of cystoids macular edema. *Am J Ophthalmol*. 2005; 140:695-702.

106. Kang SW, Sa HS, Cho HY, Kim JI. Macular grid photocoagulation after intravitreal triamcinolone acetonide for diffuse diabetic macular edema. *Arch Ophthalmol*. 2006;124:653-658.

107. Diabetic Retinopathy Clinical Research Network (DRCR. net), Beck RW, Edwards AR, et al. Three-year follow-up of a randomized trial comparing focal/grid photocoagulation and intravitreal triamcinolone for diabetic macular edema. *Arch Ophthalmol*. 2009;127:245-251.

108. Beck RW, et al. Laser-ranibizumab-triamcinolone for proliferative diabetic retinopathy. (LRTfordiabetic macular edema+PRP). NCT00445003. 2008. Clinical Trials Web site. http://www.clinicaltrials.gov. Accessed January 5, 2010

109. Maia OO Jr, Takahashi BS, Costa RA, Scott IU, Takahashi WY. Combined laser and intravitreal triamcinolone for proliferative diabetic retinopathy and macular edema: one-year results of a randomized clinical trial. *Am J Ophthalmol*. 2009;147:291-297.

110. Grant MB, Afzal A, Spoerri P, Pan H, Shaw LC, Mames RN. The role of growth factors in the pathogenesis of diabetic retinopathy. *Expert Opin Investig Drugs*. 2004;13:1275-1293.

111. Funatsu H, Yamashita H, Ikeda T, Nakanishi Y, Kitano S, Hori S. Angiotensin II and vascular endothelial growth factor in the vitreous fluid of patients with diabetic macular edema and other retinal disorders. *Am J Ophthalmol*. 2002;133:537-543.

112. Cunningham ET, Adamis AP, Aiello LP, et al. Macugen diabetic retinopathy study group. A phase II randomized double-masked trial of pegaptanib, and antivascular endothelial growth factor aptamer, for diabetic macular edema. *Ophthalmol*. 2005;112:1706-1757.

113. Chun DW, Heier JS, Topping TM, Duker JS, Bankert JM. A pilot study of multiple intravitreal injections of ranibizumab in patients with center-involving clinically significant diabetic macular edema. *Ophthalmology*. 2006;113:1706-1712.

114. Whisenant J, Bergsland E. Anti-angiogenic strategies in gastrointestinal malignancies. *Curr Treat Options Oncol*. 2005;6:411-421.

115. Kaiser PK. Antivascular endothelial growth factor agents and their development: therapeutic implications in ocular diseases. *Am J Ophthalmol*. 2006;142:660-668.

116. Lynch SS, Chen CM. Bevacizumab for neovascular ocular diseases. *Ann Pharmachother*. 2007;41:614-625.

117. Fung AE, Rosenfeld PJ, Reichel E. The international intravitreal bevacizumab safety survey: using the internet to assess drug safety worldwide. *Br J Ophthalmol*. 2006;90:1344-1349.

118. Goyal S, Lavalley M, Subramanian ML. Meta-analysis and review on the effect of bevacizumab in diabetic macular edema. *Graefes Arch Clin Exp Ophthalmol*. 2011;249:15-27.

119. Dafer RM, Schneck M, Friberg TR, Jay WM. Intravitreal ranibizumab and bevacizumab: a review of risk. *Semin Ophthalmol*. 2007;22:201-204.

120. Gillies MC. What we don't know about avastin might hurt us. *Arch Ophthalmol*. 2006; 124:1478-1479.

121. The Diabetic Retinopathy Clinical Research Network. Randomized trial evaluating ranibizumab plus or deferred laser or triamcinolone plus prompt laser for diabetic macular edema. *Ophthalmology*. 2010;117:1064-1077.

122. Efficacy and safety of ranibizumab (intravitreal injections) in patients with visual impairment due to diabetic macular edema (RESTORE). NCT00687804. Clinical Trials Web site. http://www.clinicaltrials.gov/ct2/show/NCT00687804 term_nct00687804. Accessed January 5, 2010.

123. A study of ranibizumab injection in subjects with clinically significant macular edema with center involvement secondary to diabetes mellitus (RIDE). NCT00473382. Clinical trials Web site. http://www.clinicaltrials.gov/ct2/show/NCT00473382 term_NCT00473382. Accessed January 5, 2010.

124. A study of ranibizumab injection in subjects with clinically significant macular edema with center involvement secondary to diabetes mellitus (RISE). NCT00473330. Clinical trials Web site. http://www.clinicaltrials.gov/ct2/show/NCT00473330. Accessed January 5, 2010.

8

Diabetes Mellitus and Retinal Abnormalities

Glenn C. Yiu, MD, PhD; Sandra Rocio Montezuma, MD; and Alejandro Espaillat, MD

The long-term health consequences of diabetes mellitus are an immense burden on modern health care due to the increasing incidence of obesity and sedentary lifestyle worldwide. The wide range of diabetic complications involving the ocular, renal, cardiovascular, and nervous systems are primarily attributable to the microvascular and macrovascular manifestations of the disease. In particular, diabetic retinopathy is primarily caused by retinal ischemia, exudative edema, and proliferative neovascularization. This entity has been so well studied because it is by far the most common ophthalmic complication of the disease and is also a leading cause of blindness in working-age patients in the United States.[1] Importantly, the retinal manifestations of diabetes can be readily evaluated on clinical examination without the need for costly imaging or laboratory studies. In this way, research has allowed diabetic retinopathy to be carefully quantified and used to monitor diabetes control. At the same time, the discovery of various treatment modalities from laser photocoagulation to immunopharmacology has dramatically revolutionized the management of the disease and improved the visual outcome. This chapter reviews our current understanding of diabetic retinopathy.

Epidemiology

Diabetes mellitus affects 200 million people worldwide, with 20 million in the United States alone. Diabetic retinopathy is the leading cause of new blindness in persons aged 25 to 74 years in the United States, and is continuing to rise in other parts of the world. The disease accounts for more than 8000 cases of new blindness each year.[2]

The prevalence of all types of diabetic retinopathy as well as the associated morbidity correlates with patient age and duration of diabetes. Diabetic retinopathy rarely occurs before age 10, but the risk increases after puberty and may appear as early as the second decade of life, particularly in type 1 diabetes. The Wisconsin Epidemiologic Study of Diabetic Retinopathy (WESDR), which evaluates 1210 patients with type 1 diabetes and 1780 patients with type 2 diabetes in southern Wisconsin, reported that the duration of diabetes correlates directly with the prevalence of retinopathy in both types of patients. After 20 years, nearly all patients with type 1 and >60% of those patients with type 2 diabetes have some degree of diabetic retinopathy.[3] Although the WESDR epidemiological data are limited to White patients of primarily European descent, the National Health and Nutrition Examination Survey III of patients with type 2 diabetes revealed that the

Espaillat A.
Diabetic Eye Disease: A Comprehensive Review (pp. 73-90)
© 2012 SLACK Incorporated

Table 8-1. Risk Factors for Diabetic Retinopathy	
Duration of Diabetes	Following 20 years, almost all patients with type 1 and >60% of patients with type 2 diabetes have some degree of diabetic retinopathy
HbA1c Levels	In patients with type 2 diabetes, every 1% decrease in HbA1c corresponds to 35% decrease in microvascular changes; maintenance of HbA1c <7% reduces progression of retinopathy in patients with all types of diabetes
Hypertension	Intensive blood pressure control (<150/<85 mm Hg) leads to 34% reduction in progression of diabetic retinopathy, 47% reduction in visual acuity decline, and 35% reduction in rate of laser photocoagulation compared to conventional blood pressure control (<180/<105 mm Hg).
Hyperlipidemia	Hyperlipidemia increases the risk of diabetic retinopathy and macular edema, but no relationship between serum lipids levels and progression of retinopathy has been established
Other Risk Factors	Renal disease, pregnancy, obesity, and sedentary lifestyle

Hb = hemoglobin

frequency of retinopathy is higher among non-Hispanic Blacks (27%) and Mexican Americans (33%) than in non-Hispanic Whites (18%), suggesting that race is an additional risk factor.[4]

Epidemiological studies have identified additional risk factors for developing diabetic retinopathy, including systemic hypertension, dyslipidemia, obesity, renal disease, and pregnancy. Hypertension correlates with the presence of retinopathy, most likely as a result of vascular changes associated with elevated blood pressure, which may be superimposed on the vascular manifestations of diabetes.[5] Similarly, hyperlipidemia may contribute to retinal vessel leakage and hard exudate formation.[6] The Hoorn Study, a population-based study of 2484 middle-aged Whites, revealed a positive association of retinopathy with not only elevated blood pressure, but also hypercholesterolemia, hypertriglyceridemia, and elevated body mass index (BMI) in individuals with normal or impaired glucose metabolism.[7] Nephropathy is measured by microalbuminuria and creatinine clearance, and closely correlates with the presence of retinopathy.[8] In fact, evidence suggests that aggressive management of diabetic nephropathy may have a beneficial effect on the progression of diabetic retinopathy and neovascular glaucoma. Pregnancy itself is an independent risk factor for progression of diabetic retinopathy, although the mechanism of this remains unclear (Table 8-1).[9] Less consistent risk factors associated with retinopathy in patients with diabetes include smoking[10] and physical inactivity.[11]

Diabetes imposes a tremendous economic burden to health care systems worldwide. Expenditures arising from the prevention and treatment of diabetic complications are expected to account for 11.6% of the total health care expenditures in the world in 2010-2011, which correlates to approximately 376 billion US dollars.[12] More than three-quarters of these expenditures will be used for persons who are between 50 and 80 years of age. Aside from actual medical costs, diabetes also imposes economic burdens in the form of lost productivity due to the lost value associated with disability, especially when vision is compromised. Therefore, screening and treatment paradigms for diabetic retinopathy are important to both health care and the economy.

CLINICAL EVALUATION

The onset of diabetic retinopathy often is indolent, as central visual acuity usually is preserved initially and visual symptoms develop as a late manifestation. When symptoms occur, most patients report blurry vision or distortion in their central visual field. With rare exceptions, the symptoms are slowly progressive, with little to no fluctuations.

Clinical Ophthalmoscopy

The primary methods for diagnosing diabetic retinopathy include clinical ophthalmoscopy, retinal photography, and fluorescein angiography. Ophthalmoscopy by slit-lamp evaluation using a variety of lenses is the most cost-effective way for an ophthalmologist to identify the microvascular manifestations of diabetes. Clinical instruments for examining the retina include the indirect ophthalmoscope, slit-lamp biomicroscope, and direct ophthalmoscope. All are used in a darkened room, with auxiliary handheld lenses used with indirect and slit-lamp ophthalmoscopy for viewing the posterior segment. Variations of the magnification and field of view among the different instruments allow certain features and locations of the disease to be identified. The gold standard for clinical assessment is the modified Airlie House classification, which involves the grading of 7 30-degree stereoscopic images of the retina, known as the 7 standard fields, with each image compared with standard photographs. A score is assigned to each eye, ranging from 10 (absence of retinopathy) to 85 (advanced proliferative diabetic retinopathy [PDR]), and the grades for both eyes are combined into a stepped scale. Diabetic macular edema usually is classified as either absent or present. The Diabetes Control and Complications Trial (DCCT) defined progression of diabetic retinopathy as at least 3 steps worsening from baseline,[13] whereas the United Kingdom Prospective Diabetes Study (UKPDS) defined progression as a 2-step change from baseline.[14] Telemedicine-based technology is an emerging trend in improving diabetic retinopathy screening.[15] Digital retinal images obtained at a primary care clinic can be screened remotely by an off-site ophthalmologist, reducing the need for in-person ophthalmology referral visits. Early studies show that telemedicine programs can be cost effective[16] and improve overall compliance rates.[17]

Fluorescein Angiography

Fluorescein angiography is an important imaging modality that can noticeably enhance the diagnosis of microvascular abnormalities in diabetic retinopathy. Fluorescein sodium is an orange-red crystalline hydrocarbon dye that fluoresces at a wavelength of 520 to 530 nm (green) after excitation by a light of 465 to 490 nm (blue). Photographs of the retina are taken after intravenous injection of the dye, with the first appearance in ocular circulation via the ophthalmic artery 8 to 12 seconds after the initial injection, depending on the rate of injection, patient's age, and cardiovascular status. The choroidal circulation usually is visualized first, followed by the retinal circulation due to the longer anatomical course. In diabetic retinopathy, leakage of fluorescein from retinal capillaries occurs due to compromise of the capillary endothelium. The dye is eliminated primarily through the liver and kidneys within 24 to 36 hours. Although invasive, the procedure usually is well-tolerated, with side effects including yellowish discoloration of skin or urine and mild dye hypersensitivity resulting in pruritus, rash, or rarely, anaphylaxis. Compared with clinical ophthalmoscopy, the technique can sometimes identify subtle vascular changes not easily seen on funduscopic examination, although the clinical relevance of these early changes is unclear.

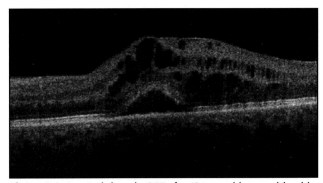

Figure 8-1. Spectral-domain OCT of a 43-year-old man with a history of diabetes mellitus type 2 for more than 10 years. The OCT reveals the presence of intraretinal cystic changes in the retina and subretinal fluid in the macula. (Reprinted with permission of Ivana Kim, MD, Massachusetts Eye and Ear Infirmary.)

Optical Coherence Tomography

Optical coherence tomography (OCT) is a noninvasive imaging modality that uses light wave coherence to generate a cross-sectional image of ocular tissues. OCT is based on imaging reflecting light, producing a 2-dimensional, false-color image of the backscattered light from different layers in the retina. The axial resolution of current commercial OCT scanners offers a resolution of 8 to 10 µm. Additional resolution may be achieved using a femtosecond titanium: sapphire laser light source, whereas Fourier-domain or spectral-domain technology can increase the speed of image capture to reduce motion artifacts (Figure 8-1). OCT is particularly useful for producing a retinal thickness map, allowing diabetic macular edema to be identified and measured in an objective manner. In this way, ophthalmologists can quantitatively monitor the progress and response of the macular edema to medical or surgical therapy.

Ultrasonography

Diagnostic ultrasonography is an invaluable tool for evaluating the posterior pole, especially when media opacities such as vitreous hemorrhage obscure the ophthalmologist's view of the fundus. Two-dimensional ultrasound imaging is known as B-scan echography, in contrast to an A-scan, which is one-dimension only. The B-scan image is a cross-sectional display of the globe and orbit with movement of the ultrasound probe allowing the examiner to create a 3-dimensional mental image (Figure 8-2). Ultrasonography allows the identification of retinal tears and detachment, among many other findings, in the posterior pole.

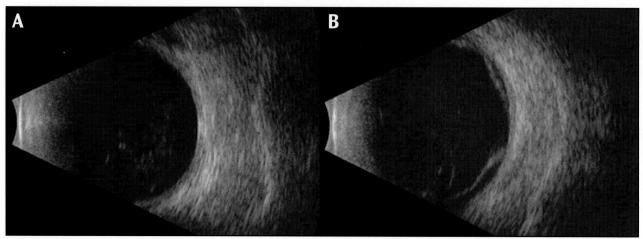

Figure 8-2. B-scan. (A) B-scan ultrasound image from a 63-year-old woman with history of diabetes for more than 10 years with decreased vision for 1 week. The patient was diagnosed with a vitreous hemorrhage, which is seen on B-scan ultrasound as low reflective mobile echoes in the vitreous cavity. The retina is attached. (B) B-scan ultrasound image from a 61-year-old woman with a history of diabetes for 14 years, who presents with decreased vision for 3 weeks. The B-scan ultrasound again shows low reflective mobile echoes in the vitreous. There is also a vitreous membrane with points of attachments causing vitreo-retinal traction. (Reprinted with permission of Ivana Kim, MD, Massachusetts Eye and Ear Infirmary.)

Laboratory Testing

Beyond imaging studies, laboratory tests allow physicians to monitor the disease severity and progress in glycemic control. Aside from blood glucose testing, glycated hemoglobin, also known as hemoglobin A1c (HbA1c), is an important measure of a patient's glycemic control over the previous 3-month period. Early epidemiologic studies have shown a consistent relationship between HbA1c levels and the incidence of diabetic retinopathy[18]; this was later confirmed in large randomized controlled studies including the DCCT[19] and UKPDS.[20] In patients with type 2 diabetes, every 1% decrease in HbA1c is associated with 35% reduction in microvascular endpoints, and 17% reduction in all-cause mortality.[14] In this way, close monitoring of glycemic control is important not only for assessing the risk for onset or progression of diabetic retinopathy, but also for long-term management of the diabetes itself.

CLASSIFICATION

Diabetic retinopathy is classified into an early non-proliferative stage and a more advanced proliferative stage. Nonproliferative diabetic retinopathy (NPDR) is characterized by microvascular changes of retinal circulation, including the appearance of microaneurysms, small intraretinal hemorrhages, nerve fiber layer infarctions known as cotton-wool spots, and venous beading. Exudative extravasation from the retinal capillary beds in the macula leads to diabetic macular edema, which accounts for the majority of the visual impairment resulting from diabetic retinopathy. NPDR is sometimes referred to as background diabetic retinopathy (BDR) and may be classified as mild, moderate, severe, or very severe.

PDR occurs when the ischemia associated with these microvascular changes induces the abnormal growth of new vessels, a process known as neovascularization. Neovascular disease may occur in the retina, optic disc, iris, or angle of the anterior chamber. PDR may be categorized as non-high risk and high risk. The pathogenesis, evaluation, and management of NPDR and PDR will be discussed separately in the following sections.

Nonproliferative Diabetic Retinopathy

Pathogenesis

Diabetic retinopathy is primarily a manifestation of the microvascular damage resulting from chronic hyperglycemia. The progression of diabetic retinopathy correlates to the severity and duration of hyperglycemia and may also be associated with the vasculopathy induced by hypertension and hyperlipidemia as well. However, the exact mechanism by which hyperglycemia leads to vascular injury remains unclear. Molecular models that have been postulated for the pathogenesis of diabetic retinopathy include accumulation of polyols and advanced glycosylation end-products (AGEs), oxidative stress, as well as growth hormones, growth factors, and their downstream signaling pathways.

Animal studies showed that prolonged hyperglycemia leads to the accumulation of polyols, such as sorbitol, via the enzymatic activity of aldose reductase.

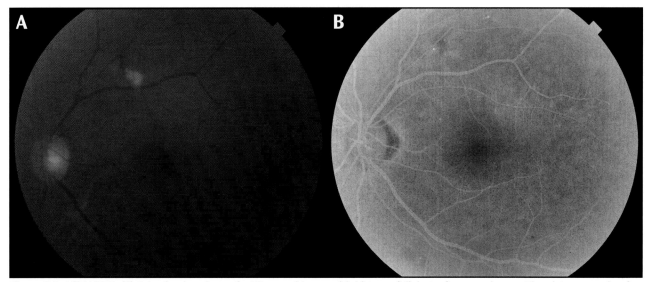

Figure 8-3. Mild NPDR. (A) Color fundus photo of a 58-year-old man with history of diabetes for several years. The picture reveals a few small microaneurisms, and a white patch along the superior temporal arcade consistent with a cotton wool spot. (B) The fluorescein angiogram at 1 minute demonstrates a few pinpoint hyperfluorescent spots corresponding to microaneurisms and a small area of hypofluorescence along the superior temporal arcade corresponding to the cotton wool spot. (Reprinted with permission of Demetrios G. Vavvas, MD, Massachusetts Eye and Ear Infirmary.)

The increase in sorbitol concentration has been hypothesized to result in osmotic damage to retinal vascular endothelial cells, specifically resulting in the loss of pericytes and thickening of the basement membrane.[21,22] Elevated blood glucose also results in formation of AGEs by nonenzymatic binding of glucose to protein side chains, which can lead to microaneurysm formation and pericyte loss.[23,24]

Oxidative stress is believed to arise due to the formation of reactive oxygen species in the setting of chronic hyperglycemia.[25] Normalization of glucose-induced superoxide production decreases the vascular damage caused by hyperglycemia.[26] Importantly, studies have demonstrated that antioxidants such as vitamin E may prevent some of the vascular dysfunction associated with diabetes.[27,28]

Research in understanding the biochemical pathways involved in diabetic retinopathy has revealed the involvement of a number of growth factors, such as vascular endothelial growth factor (VEGF),[29] and growth hormones, such as insulin-like growth factor-1 (IGF-1).[30] An important signaling mediator of these pathways is diacylglycerol and its downstream target, protein kinase C (PKC). Activation of PKC causes cellular changes, leading to enhanced permeability of retinal vasculature, alterations in retinal blood flow, and basement membrane thickening.[31] Together, these changes trigger the microvascular dysfunction that leads to diabetic retinopathy.

The earliest manifestation of diabetic retinopathy is the formation of microaneurysms, tiny outpouchings of retinal vessels due to weakening of capillary vessel walls. With time, fibrin and erythrocytes may accumulate in their lumen. Eventual rupture of microaneurysms leads to intraretinal hemorrhages. As retinal ischemia progresses, venous beading and venous loops may occur. Infarctions of the superficial nerve fiber layer lead to blockage of axoplasmic flow in retinal ganglion cell axons, leading to the formation of cotton-wool spots (Figure 8-3). Persistent hypoxia also triggers remodeling of retinal vessels to act as shunts across areas of nonperfusion. This nonproliferative form of vessel remodeling occurs through endothelial cell proliferation and results in intraretinal microvascular abnormalities (IRMA). With progression of NPDR, visual function is eventually affected by 2 mechanisms—macular edema and macular ischemia.

Macular edema occurs with increased compromise of the retinal capillary walls and breakdown of the blood-retinal barrier, which allow fluids and proteins to leak from the microvasculature into the extracellular space. Such leakage leads to focal hard exudates as well as retinal edema. When this edematous thickening occurs in the macula, decreased central vision may occur. In fact, macular edema is the most common cause of vision loss in patients with NPDR.

Macular ischemia is a result of progressive retinal capillary nonperfusion. The foveal avascular zone (FAZ) may become enlarged or irregular due to poor perfusion of the marginal capillaries. Over time, retinal ischemia can promote the release of vasoproliferative factors to stimulate new vessel formation. The onset of neovascularization delineates the progression of NPDR to PDR. The pathogenesis of PDR will be more thoroughly addressed in the second part of this chapter.

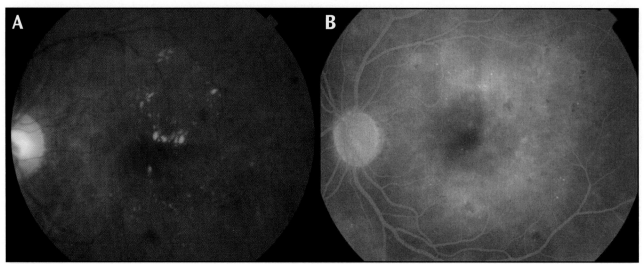

Figure 8-4. Clinical significant macular edema. (A) Color fundus photo of a 69-year-old woman with a history of diabetes for 17 years. The picture reveals multiple hard exudates located within 500 µm of center of the Foveal Avascular Zone (FAZ) with adjacent retinal thickening. (B) The fluorescein angiography reveals diffuse leakage of the macula and pinpoint areas of hyperfluorescence corresponding to microaneurysms. (Reprinted with permission of Lucy H. Young, MD, Massachusetts Eye and Ear Infirmary.)

Clinical Features

Early signs of diabetic retinopathy include microaneurysms and intraretinal hemorrhages. Microaneurysms appear as small red dots in the superficial retinal layers, most often adjacent to vessels. They may appear yellowish with time as endothelial cells proliferate and produce basement membrane. As microaneurysms rupture in the deeper layers of the retina, such as the inner nuclear and outer plexiform layers, small intraretinal hemorrhages known as dot (very small) and blot (small) hemorrhages form. Clinically, they appear similar to microaneurysms and may be difficult to distinguish without the use of fluorescein angiography. Splinter hemorrhages occur in the superficial layers of the retina and are readily recognizable by their conformation to the contour of the nerve fiber layer. Infarction of the nerve fiber layer leads to cotton-wool spots, which appear as fluffy white patches in the superficial retina, often bordered by microaneurysms and vascular hyperpermeability. On fluorescein angiography, cotton-wool spots may correspond to areas of capillary nonperfusion. Venous beading and venous loops may also be seen adjacent to these areas. Intraretinal microvascular abnormalities are remodeled capillary beds with no proliferative changes or leakage on fluorescein angiography.

Diabetic Macular Edema

Macular edema is the leading cause of visual impairment in patients with diabetes. Interestingly, diabetic macular edema is more common in type 2 than in type 1 diabetes.[2] In fact, although PDR is the most common sight-threatening lesion in patients with type 1

diabetes, macular edema is the primary cause of poor visual acuity in patients with type 2 diabetes. Clinically significant macular edema (CSME) was first defined in the Early Treatment of Diabetic Retinopathy Study (ETDRS), a randomized clinical trial designed to evaluate laser photocoagulation and aspirin treatment in the management of NPDR or early PDR. The study showed that focal laser therapy is indicated for CSME, which is defined as any of the following:

- Retinal thickening within 500 µm of center of the FAZ.
- Hard exudates within 500 µm of the center of the FAZ with adjacent retinal thickening (Figure 8-4).
- Retinal thickening 1 disc area or larger in size located within 1 disc diameter of the FAZ.

Staging

Staging of NPDR is classified by the International Clinical Diabetic Retinopathy Disease Severity Scale. NPDR may be mild, moderate, severe, or very severe. Mild NPDR is characterized by the presence of microaneurysms only (Figure 8-5). Moderate NPDR usually involves the presence of not only microaneurysms, but also intraretinal hemorrhages (dot and blot hemorrhages) and hard exudates (Figure 8-6). Soft exudates, venous beading, and IRMAs are sometimes present as well. Severe NPDR is diagnosed if the patient meets one of the following criteria (Figure 8-7):

- Retinal hemorrhages and microaneurysms in all 4 quadrants
- Venous beading in at least 2 quadrants.
- IRMA in at least 1 quadrant.

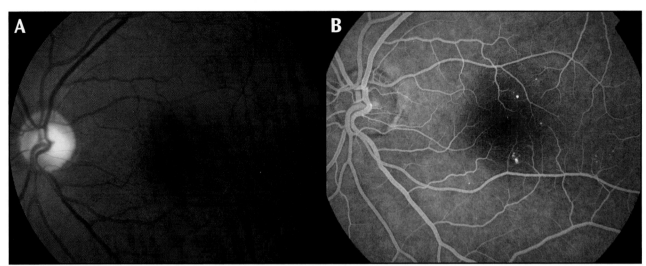

Figure 8-5. Mild NPDR. (A) Color fundus photo of a 66-year-old man with a history of diabetes for more than 6 years. The picture shows small microaneurisms. (B) The fluorescein angiogram at 1 minute reveals pinpoint spots of hyperfluorescence, corresponding to these microaneurysms. (Reprinted with permission of Lucy H. Young, MD, Massachusetts Eye and Ear Infirmary.)

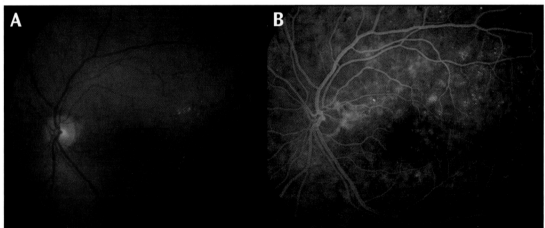

Figure 8-6. Moderate NPDR. (A) Color fundus photo of a 67-year-old man with a history of diabetes for 30 years, showing microaneurisms, hard exudates, and small dot hemorrhages in the macula. There are dot and blot hemorrhages superiorly. (B) The fluorescein angiogram at 1 minute show small hyperfluorescent microaneurysms and blockage of the fluorescence in the areas of hemorrhage. There is also diffuse macular edema. (Reprinted with permission of Lucy H. Young, MD, Massachusetts Eye and Ear Infirmary.)

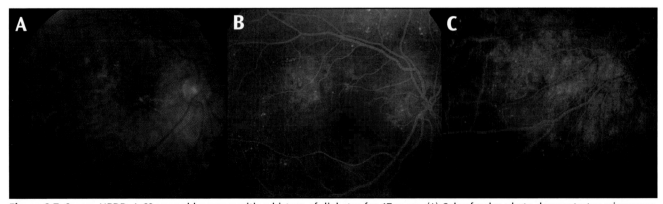

Figure 8-7. Severe NPDR. A 69-year-old woman with a history of diabetes for 17 years. (A) Color fundus photo demonstrates microaneurysms and dot and blot hemorrhages in the temporal macula and outside the vascular arcades. Retinal hemorrhages are present in all 4 quadrants. (B) The fluorescein angiogram shows hyperfluorescence of the microaneurysms in the posterior pole. Superotemporal to the macula, there is a patch of hyperfluorescence corresponding to leakage and macular edema.(C) There are areas of capillary nonperfusion and microaneurysms in the nasal periphery of the other eye. These findings are present in all 4 quadrants. (Reprinted with permission of Ivana Kim, MD, Massachusetts Eye and Ear Infirmary.)

Table 8-2. Staging of Diabetic Retinopathy

NPDR

Mild NPDR	Microaneurysm only
Moderate NPDR	Microaneurysm, intraretinal hemorrhage, and exudates
Severe NPDR	Any of the following features: a) intraretinal hemorrhages and microaneurysms in all 4 quadrants; b) venous beading in at least 2 quadrants; c) IRMA
Very severe NPDR	Two of the criteria for severe NPDR

PDR

Mild risk PDR	Any presence of neovascularization that does not meet the criteria for high-risk PDR
High-risk PDR	Any of the following features: a) NVD >1/3 disc area; b) any NVD with vitreous or preretinal hemorrhage; c) NVE >1/2 disc area with vitreous or preretinal

NPDR = nonproliferative diabetic retinopathy, IRMA = intraretinal vascular abnormalities, PDR = proliferative diabetic retinopathy, NVD = neovascularization of the disc, NVE = neovascularization elsewhere

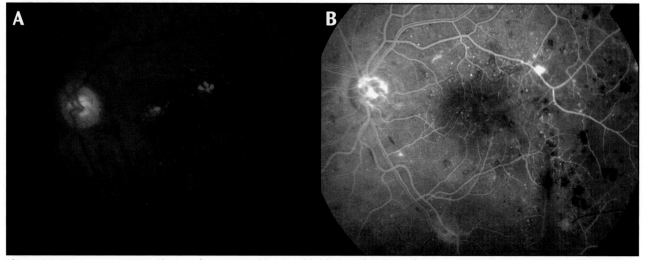

Figure 8-8. Very severe NPDR. Picture of a 49-year-old man with history of diabetes for more than 10 years. (A) Color fundus photo reveals multiple exudates and microaneurisms. There are dot and blot hemorrhages in all 4 quadrants and intraretinal microvascular abnormalities (IRMA) in the temporal macula. (B) The fluorescein angiogram at 40 seconds shows mutiple small hyperfluorescent microaneurisms in the macula. There is focal blockage of the fluorescence in the areas of hemorrhage, hyperfluorescence of the IRMA in the temporal macula, and mild hyperfluourescence of the optic nerve. There are also areas of capillary nonperfusion inferiorly and temporally. (Reprinted with permission of Lucy H. Young, MD, Massachusetts Eye and Ear Infirmary.)

This classification scheme was developed also as part of the ETDRS to help clinicians identify patients who are at greatest risk for progression to PDR (Table 8-2). The study showed that severe NPDR had a 15% chance of progression to high-risk PDR within 1 year, whereas very severe NPDR, defined by the presence of 2 of the listed criteria, had a 45% chance of progression to high-risk PDR within 1 year (Figure 8-8).[32]

Management

Glycemic Control

The primary medical intervention to minimize long-term complications in diabetes is glucose control. The DCCT, a multicenter, randomized clinical trial of 1441 patients with type 1 diabetes comparing intensive with conventional diabetes therapy, demonstrated that intensive glucose control reduced the incidence of diabetic retinopathy by 76% and progression of retinopathy by 54% compared with conventional treatment.[13,33,34] Similarly, the UKPDS, another multicenter randomized trial of 3867 newly diagnosed patients with type 2 diabetes, showed that intensive therapy reduced microvascular end points by 25% and the need for laser photocoagulation by 29%.[14] Together, these 2 studies support the importance of tight glycemic control, with maintenance of glycosylated hemoglobin levels of <7% to limit retinopathy in all types of patients with diabetes.

Interestingly, long-term observational data from the DCCT showed that despite equalization of HbA1c values after termination of the study, the rate of retinopathy progression in the former intensive treatment group remained significantly lower than the former conventional treatment group, suggesting that tight glycemic control early in the course of the disease may have persistent benefits in the long term.[33,35] Nevertheless, intensive glycemic control may also be associated with significant adverse effects, including hypoglycemic episodes and diabetic ketoacidosis.[36] A meta-analysis of 14 randomized controlled trials, including the DCCT, showed that intensive treatment is associated with a 3-fold risk of hypoglycemia and 70% higher risk of ketoacidosis compared with conventional treatment.[37] These reports suggest that glucose control in patients with diabetes should be tailored to individual cases.

Blood Pressure Control

In addition to glycemic control, blood pressure is another important modifiable risk factor for diabetic retinopathy. The UKPDS randomized 1048 patients with hypertension to tight blood pressure control (<150/<85 mm Hg) or conventional control (<180/<105 mm Hg), and showed that patients under intensive blood pressure control had a 34% reduction in progression of diabetic retinopathy, a 47% reduction in visual acuity decline, and a 35% reduction in rate of laser photocoagulation compared to conventional blood pressure targets.[38] In contrast, the Appropriate Blood Pressure Control in Diabetes (ABCD) trial, a randomized study of 470 patients with type 2 diabetes with hypertension, showed no difference in the progression of diabetic retinopathy between intensive or moderate blood pressure control.[39] However, the study is limited by poorer glycemic control and shorter follow-up compared with the UKPDS. Surprisingly, antihypertensive therapy is also beneficial in normotensive individuals. A second arm of the ABCD study included 480 normotensive type 2 diabetics and demonstrated a significant reduction in retinopathy progression with tight blood pressure control compared to moderate control.[40]

More recent clinical studies using specific antihypertensive agents, particularly those that disrupt the renin-angiotensin system, have also showed similar benefits. Mounting evidence suggests that activation of the renin-angiotensin system may play an important role in the pathogenesis of diabetic retinopathy, with major components of the pathway being overexpressed in the diabetic retina.[41] Pharmacological blockade at the level of angiotensin-converting enzyme (ACE) or angiotensin II (AT) receptors has specifically been shown to reduce VEGF concentrations.[41] The EURODIAB Controlled Trial of Lisinopril in Insulin-Dependent Diabetes Mellitus (EUCLID) demonstrated that normotensive type 1 diabetic patients taking the ACE inhibitor lisinopril showed a significant 50% reduction in

progression of diabetic retinopathy. However, the study was confounded by lower baseline glycemic levels in the treatment group and a short follow-up of 2 years. In fact, the Diabetic Retinopathy Candesartan Trials (DIRECT), which evaluated the AT-receptor antagonist candesartan compared with placebo, showed only a nonsignificant reduction in primary prevention and no difference for secondary prevention in patients with type 1 diabetes,[42] and a nonsignificant reduction in secondary prevention in patients with type 2 diabetes.[43] The Action in Diabetes and Vascular Disease (ADVANCE) study, which evaluates patients with type 2 diabetes taking an ACE inhibitor-diuretic combination (perindopril-indapamide), also showed no significant benefit to the incidence or progression of diabetic retinopathy when compared with placebo. Furthermore, data from the UKPDS[44] or ABCD study[39] did not show superiority of any specific medications such as ACE inhibitors over other antihypertensive agents. Therefore, although blood pressure control plays an important role in limiting diabetic retinopathy, there are insufficient data to support the use of any specific antihypertensive agent.

Lipid-Lowering Therapy

Elevated lipid levels in systemic circulation are associated with vasculopathy and are another potentially modifiable risk factor for diabetic retinopathy. Indeed, some observational studies suggest that hyperlipidemia may be associated with an increased risk of retinopathy, particularly macular edema.[7,45] The Fenofibrate Intervention and Event Lowering in Diabetes (FIELD) study showed that fenofibrate reduced progression of diabetic retinopathy and need for laser therapy in 9795 patients with type 2 diabetes.[46] However, no relationship between serum lipids and the onset or progression of retinopathy was demonstrated. Fenofibrate is a peroxisome proliferator-activated receptor (PPAR)-g agonist used primarily for the treatment of hypertriglyceridemia, but it is also effective in lowering total and low-density lipoprotein cholesterol and increasing high-density lipoprotein cholesterol. It is uncertain, therefore, whether the benefit arises from the lipid-lowering effect of the drug. In fact, the Collaborative Atorvastatin Diabetes Study (CARDS), another randomized controlled trial of 2830 patients with type 2 diabetes, did not find atorvastatin to be effective in reducing the progression of diabetic retinopathy.[47] The ongoing ACCORD-EYE study will evaluate the effects of lipid control using statins alone versus statins with fenofibrate on diabetic retinopathy.[48]

Anti-Platelet Therapy

The ETDRS demonstrated no additional benefit from 650 mg of aspirin daily on visual acuity loss or progression of diabetic retinopathy in patients with diabetic macular edema or severe NPDR.[49] However, aspirin use significantly reduces morbidity and mortality arising from cardiovascular complications in diabetic patients and is not associated with an increased rate of vitreous hemorrhage.[49] Hence, although aspirin use is not routinely recommended specifically for the prevention of diabetic retinopathy, it is not contraindicated from an ophthalmologic standpoint. A recent randomized controlled trial evaluating aspirin alone and in combination with dipyridamole reported a reduction in microaneurysms on fluorescein angiograms in both groups when compared to placebo.[50] The clinical relevance of these findings, however, remains uncertain.

Other Medical Therapy

Recent research in understanding the pathogenesis of diabetic retinopathy has revealed new hormonal, enzymatic, or signaling targets for medical therapy. Increased levels of insulin-like growth factor have been associated with severe diabetic retinopathy.[51] Octreotide, a synthetic analog of somatostatin, which blocks growth hormone, has yet to be found to have significant benefits in randomized trials.[52] Pharmacological inhibitors of aldose reductase, a rate-limiting enzyme in glucose metabolism, have also had no significant effect in reducing the onset or progression of diabetic retinopathy.[53] Another drug target has been PKC, a signaling intermediate triggered by hyperglycemia and known to be involved in the pathogenesis of diabetic retinopathy. However, neither the Protein Kinase C Diabetic Retinopathy Study (PKC-DRS,[54] PKC-DRS2[55]) or the Protein Kinase C Diabetic Macular Edema Study (PKC-DMES[56]), which evaluated the use of the PKC-inhibitor ruboxistaurin, showed any significant benefit in progression of diabetic retinopathy or incidence of diabetic macular edema, respectively. Future advances will yield new therapeutic targets in the treatment of diabetic retinopathy.

Laser Photocoagulation

Laser photocoagulation was developed in the 1960s, allowing the delivery of highly focused light energy to create a coagulative response in target tissues. In patients with CSME, focal laser photocoagulation may be delivered directly to treat leaking vessels or microaneurysms causing the edema, or grid pattern laser can be used to treat diffuse leakage or zones of nonperfusion. Focal laser treatment is applied as 50- to 100-μm spots, <0.1 second in duration, to all leaking microaneurysms between 500 and 3000 μm from the center of the macula, with the goal of whitening or darkening the microaneurysms. For grid laser treatment, a grid pattern of 50- to 100-μm spots, <0.1 second in duration, spaced at least 1 burn width apart, is applied to all areas of diffuse leakage more than 500 μm from the center of the macula and 500 μm from the temporal margin of the optic disc.[57]

The efficacy of focal laser photocoagulation in diabetic macular edema was first evaluated in the ETDRS. The results showed that focal laser surgery reduces the incidence of moderate visual loss (defined as doubling of the visual angle or approximately loss of 2 lines of Snellen visual acuity) from 30% to 15% over a 3-year period when compared to observation alone.[58] Favorable prognostic factors include circular exudates of recent onset, well-defined areas of leakage, and good perifoveal perfusion. Poor prognostic factors include diffuse macular edema, diffuse fluorescein leakage, macular ischemia, hard exudates in the fovea, and significant cystoid macular edema.[58] No clear evidence supports that any specific laser type (argon, diode, dye, krypton) is superior over the others. Adverse effects include inadvertent foveal burn, color vision loss, and retinal fibrosis. It is important to emphasize to patients that focal or grid laser treatment is not aimed at improving vision, but rather at reducing the risk of moderate visual loss.

The ETDRS also evaluated the use of early panretinal photocoagulation (PRP) in decreasing the risk of diabetic retinopathy progression. PRP is another form of laser therapy that, unlike focal or grid laser, involves the widespread placement of laser burns over the entire retina, sparing the central macula. In the study, early PRP treatment decreased the risk of progression to high-risk PDR by 50% as compared with deferral, although the incidence of severe visual loss (<5/200 for at least 4 months) was low in both groups.[59] However, early PRP was not shown to be beneficial in mild or moderate NPDR and may be most effective in patients with type 2 diabetes. Additional details regarding PRP treatment will be discussed in the section on the management of PDR.

Vitreoretinal Surgery

Diffuse macular edema that is poorly responsive to focal laser therapy may benefit from vitreoretinal surgery. Vitrectomy is a surgical procedure where the vitreous is removed through microsurgical techniques, eliminating vitreous traction on the macula and helping reduce macular edema. However, the few randomized trials are small, have short follow-up, and produced inconsistent results. Although 2 studies showed reduced macular thickness and improved visual acuity after vitrectomy compared to observation[60] and superiority over laser therapy,[61] others showed no such benefit to surgery.[62] Furthermore, vitreoretinal procedures are associated with a significant risk of complications, including recurrent vitreous hemorrhage, retinal tears and detachment, cataract formation, and glaucoma. As a result, vitrectomy should be reserved for recalcitrant cases for which vitreous traction is documented on OCT.

Intravitreal Corticosteroids

Due to their potent anti-inflammatory and anti-angiogenesis effects, corticosteroids may be indicated for either diabetic macular edema or PDR. Due to the significant side effects associated with systemic corticosteroid use, most resulting from suppression of the hypopituitary-pituitary-adrenal axis, intraocular delivery of corticosteroids has been the mainstay for the treatment of diabetic macular edema. A randomized controlled study has shown that an intravitreal injection of triamcinolone acetonide (4 mg) produced a significant decrease in macular edema and increased probability of visual acuity improvement compared to placebo injections.[63] However, recent reports from the DRCR.net showed that despite some reduction in CSME, the effect of intravitreal triamcinolone is not as effective as focal or grid laser treatment at the primary endpoint of 2 years.[64] Moreover, steroid injections also significantly increased the risk of intraocular pressure elevation, infection, and cataract formation. The procedure is invasive, requires a skilled specialist, and must be frequently repeated to maintain an adequate intraocular level of the drug.

Recently, intravitreal and retinal implants have been developed for extended delivery of corticosteroids. A randomized trial using the surgically implanted intravitreal fluocinolone acetonide (Retisert) demonstrated improvement in diabetic macular edema and visual acuity, but also showed a significantly higher risk of glaucoma and cataract formation, with 5% of patients requiring implant removal for control of elevated intraocular pressure.[65] Another study using an injectable intravitreal dexamethasone implant (Posurdex, Allergan, Irvine, CA) showed similar improvement in macular edema and visual acuity, although the study had short follow-up and included macular edema from other causes such as retinal vein occlusion, uveitis, and cataract surgery.[65] Further studies are required to assess the long-term efficacy and safety of intravitreal corticosteroid delivery.

Intravitreal Anti-Angiogenesis Therapy

VEGF has been known to play an important role in the pathogenesis of diabetic retinopathy. Similar to corticosteroids, anti-VEGF therapy has the potential to reduce vascular permeability and neovascularization, important features of diabetic macular edema and PDR, respectively. Anti-VEGF agents also require intraocular delivery due to the potentially devastating side effects of systemic inhibition of angiogenesis, which can affect the vascular response to ischemia in diabetic patients with cardiovascular, cerebrovascular, or peripheral vascular disease. Currently, 3 anti-VEGF agents are available, including pegaptanib sodium (Macugen), ranibizumab (Lucentis), and bevacizumab (Avastin). Aflibercept (VEGF Trap-Eye) is not yet available.

Pegaptanib is a PEGylated (ie, conjugated to polyethylene glycol) neutralizing ribonucleic acid aptamer with a high affinity for the 165 isoform of VEGF, which is believed to be the isoform involved in pathologic, and not physiologic, neovascularization. Aptamers are single-stranded nucleic acids that bind to specific targets but do not exhibit immunogenicity like antibodies. A randomized controlled trial of 172 patients with diabetic macular edema showed that repeated intravitreal pegaptanib yielded improved visual acuity, reduced retinal thickness, and decreased the need for additional focal laser treatment at 36 weeks compared to placebo injections.[66]

Ranibizumab is a fragment of a recombinant humanized monoclonal antibody against VEGF, and unlike pegaptanib, inhibits all isoforms of human VEGF. It was approved by the US Food and Drug Administration (FDA) for neovascular age-related macular degeneration (AMD) in 2006. Bevacizumab is the full-length, monoclonal anti-VEGF antibody, which was approved by the FDA in 2004 for the treatment of metastatic colorectal cancer. It is not licensed for intraocular use, but has been used off-label as intravitreal injections for treatment of neovascular AMD due to its lower cost. To date, uncontrolled studies using ranibizumab and bevacizumab have shown some promise, although a comparison of intravitreal bevacizumab with intravitreal triamcinolone showed greater improvements in foveal thickness and visual outcomes than corticosteroids.[67] Current randomized controlled trials are under way to evaluate the efficacy of ranibizumab[68,69] and bevacizumab[70] in diabetic macular edema.

Aflibercept is a fusion protein composed of extracellular domain segments of VEGF-receptors 1 and 2 fused to the constant region of human immunoglobulin G. It has a higher binding affinity and longer duration of action than other anti-VEGF agents. It is currently under evaluation in a phase 2 randomized study.[71]

Follow-Up

The long-term management of diabetic retinopathy requires regular monitoring of progression and early intervention when necessary. The frequency of follow-up is determined primarily by the stage of retinopathy and the associated rate of progression to PDR. Patients with mild NPDR have a 5% chance of progression to PDR within 1 year and should thus be evaluated every 6 to 12 months. Those with moderate NPDR have a 27% probability of progression to PDR within 1 year and are seen every 4 to 8 months. For severe NPDR, >50% of patients progress to PDR within 1 year and require more frequent monitoring up to every 2 to 4 months. If CSME is present, the patient should be seen every 2 to 3 months regardless of the stage of NPDR.[72]

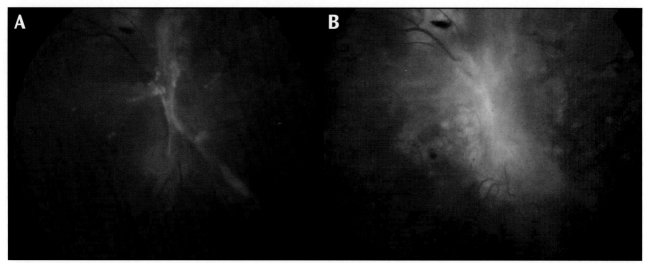

Figure 8-9. PDR with neovascularization of the disc. Picture of a 49-year-old man with a history of diabetes for more than 10 years. (A) Color picture reveals a fibrovascular proliferation over the optic nerve head and some dot and blot hemorrhages in the macula and superior to the optic nerve. (B) Late frames of the fluorescein angiogram reveal hyperfluorescence of the optic nerve head showing fibrovascular proliferation with diffuse leakage. (Reprinted with permission of John Loewenstein, MD, Massachusetts Eye and Ear Infirmary.)

Proliferative Diabetic Retinopathy

Pathogenesis

PDR is defined by the appearance of neovascularization of the retina or optic disc. As NPDR evolves, the progressive increase in retinal ischemia leads to the production of vasoproliferative factors, such as VEGF, that stimulate new vessel formation.[29] Extracellular matrix degradation occurs through the action of proteases, and new abnormal vessels arising primarily from retinal venules can penetrate the internal limiting membrane and form capillary networks between the inner surface of the retina and posterior hyaloid face. Neovascularization usually appears at the borders of perfused and nonperfused retina, most commonly along the vascular arcades and at the optic nerve head. These vessels often are friable and highly permeable, predisposing them to leakage or damage, resulting in hemorrhage.

The 2 primary sequelae of high-risk PDR are vitreous hemorrhage and traction retinal detachment. Vitreous hemorrhage occurs when the fragile neovascular vessels bleed, causing hemorrhage into the vitreous cavity, preretinal, or intraretinal space. In later stages, as new vessels grow and older vessels regress, fibrovascular scarring can develop and become adherent to both the retina and posterior hyaloid face. Vitreous contraction may exert tractional forces across these fibroglial connections, resulting in retinal tears and traction retinal detachment.

Clinical Features

The hallmark of PDR is the presence of neovascularization. Neovascularization of the disc (NVD) appears as fine vessels overlying the optic nerve head (Figure 8-9), whereas neovascularization elsewhere (NVE) appears as networks of thin vessels in the retina, which usually occur within 3 disc diameters of major retinal vessels (Figure 8-10). On fluorescein angiography, these abnormal vessels are highly permeable and prone to dye leakage. They start as hyperfluorescent areas in early phases and continue to increase in size and intensity in later phases of the angiogram (Figure 8-11).

Hemorrhages from neovascular vessels can occur in the retina (intraretinal), in the potential space between the retina and posterior hyaloid face (subhyaloid), or in the vitreous cavity (vitreal). Intraretinal hemorrhages tend to appear as irregular patches or spots, or may conform to the contour of the nerve fiber layer as splinter hemorrhages. Subhyaloid hemorrhages often show pooling and appear boat-shaped, depending on the amount and shape of the subhyaloid space. Vitreous hemorrhages are poorly circumscribed, appear as diffuse haze or clumps of blood clots, and often settle inferiorly due to gravity (Figure 8-12). When the media is opacified by the presence of vitreous blood, B-scan ultrasonography is an important tool for evaluating the posterior pole.

Fibrovascular proliferation often is associated with the neovascular complex and may appear avascular if the vessels have regressed. Traction retinal detachments usually are tented, immobile, and concave (Figure 8-13). This contrasts with rhegmatogenous retinal detachment resulting from retinal tears or holes, which has a bullous, mobile, and convex appearance.

Neovascularization can also occur in the anterior segment, including both the iris (NVI) and anterior chamber angle (NVA). The mechanism is believed to arise from angiogenic factors diffusing from the ischemic

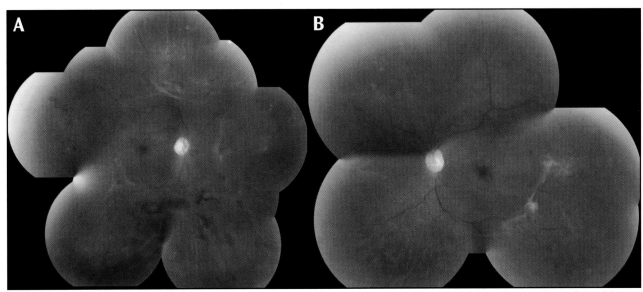

Figure 8-10. PDR. Picture of a 50-year-old man with a history of diabetes for more than 15 years. (A) The fundus photo of the right eye shows pre-retinal fibrovascular proliferation along the vascular arcades and nasal retina associated with a tractional retinal detachment. There is preretinal hemorrhage in the inferior retina, with dot and blot hemorrhage in all 4 quadrants and IRMA in the temporal mid-periphery. (B) The photo of the left eye demonstrates pre-retinal fibrovascular proliferation along the inferotemporal vascular arcade, with attenuation of the vessels, as well as dot and blot hemorrhages in all 4 quadrants. (Reprinted with permission of Ivana Kim, MD, Massachusetts Eye and Ear Infirmary.)

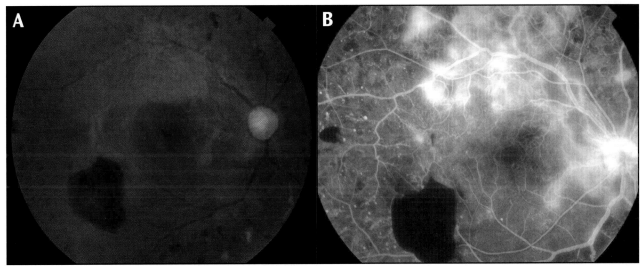

Figure 8-11. PDR. Picture of a 51-year-old woman with a history of diabetes for more than 12 years. (A) The color fundus photo demonstrates a fibrous neovascular frond superiorly, and a patch of pre-retinal hemorrhage inferiorly. There is tortuosity and venous beading of the superotemporal vessels, and multiple round laser scars. (B) The fluorescein angiogram at 1 minute reveals diffuse hyperfluorescence of the optic nerve and superotemporal vessels, with blockage of fluorescence in the areas of hemorrhage. There are also multiple small microaneurysms. (Reprinted with permission of John Loewenstein, MD, Massachusetts Eye and Ear Infirmary.)

retina into anterior segment structures. When significant neovascularization occurs at these locations, hemorrhage may occur in the anterior chamber or a neovascular glaucoma may ensue (Figure 8-14). Acute elevation of intraocular pressure in the setting of angle neovascularization requires prompt PRP treatment or anti-VEGF therapy in addition to standard topical treatment.

Staging

PDR is grossly classified as non–high-risk PDR or high-risk PDR. High-risk PDR was described in the Diabetic Retinopathy Study (DRS) to help ophthalmologists assess the indication for PRP and is defined as any of the following (see Table 8-2):

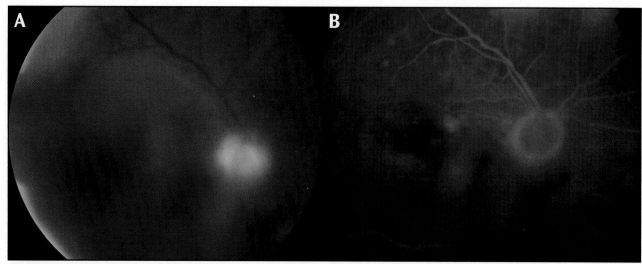

Figure 8-12. PDR with vitreous hemorrhage. (A) Color fundus photo of a 65-year-old man with a history of diabetes for more than 20 years. The color picture reveals vitreous hemorrhage. (B) The fluorescein angiogram shows corresponding blockage of the retina view in the areas of vitreous hemorrhage. (Reprinted with permission of John Loewenstein, MD, Massachusetts Eye and Ear Infirmary.)

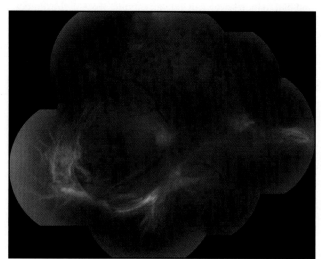

Figure 8-13. PDR with tractional retinal detachment. Color fundus photo of a 60-year-old man with history of diabetes for more than 30 years. Color picture reveals a fibrovascular proliferation of the inferior retina with areas of tractional retinal detachment. There are multiple laser scars superiorly. (Reprinted with permission of Lucy H. Young, MD, Massachusetts Eye and Ear Infirmary.)

- NVD greater than one-third of the disc area
- Any NVD with vitreous or preretinal hemorrhage.
- NVE greater than or equal to half the disc area with vitreous or preretinal hemorrhage

Non–high-risk PDR is any presence of neovascularization that does not meet the criteria for high-risk PDR. Based on the DRS results, the presence of high-risk PDR is an indication for immediate treatment with PRP.

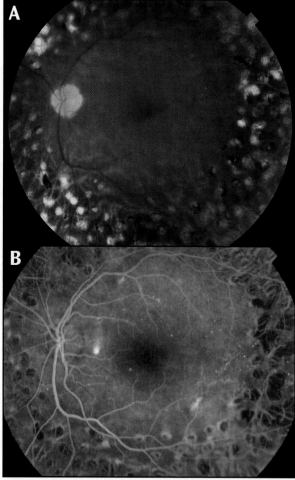

Figure 8-14. PDR status post panretinal photocoagulation (PRP). (A) Color fundus photo of a 39-year-old man with a history of type 1 diabetes for more than 20 years, demonstrating multiple mid-peripheral round laser scars. (B) The fluorescein angiogram at one minute reveals multiple hypofluorescent small round lesions with a hyperfluorescent halo, consistent with retinal laser scars. (Reprinted with permission of Shizuo Mukai, MD, Massachusetts Eye and Ear Infirmary.)

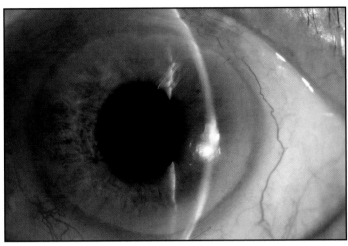

Figure 8-15. PDR with neovascular glaucoma, status post Ahmed Glaucoma Valve (New World Medical, Inc., Rancho Cucamonga, CA) placement. Picture of an 84-year-old man with a history of diabetes for more than 22 years, history of proliferative diabetic retinopathy, and multiple panretinal photocoagulation treatments. Despite multiple laser treatments, the patient developed neovascular glaucoma of the right eye. Color slit lamp photos reveals neovascularization of the iris and the presence of a tube in the anterior chamber corresponding to the glaucoma valve. (Reprinted with permission of Joan Miller, MD, Massachusetts Eye and Ear Infirmary.)

Management

As in NPDR, management of PDR requires intensive glycemic and blood pressure control, as demonstrated in the DCCT for type 1 diabetics and in the UKPDS for patients with type 2 diabetes. Current recommendations by the American Diabetes Association (ADA) support the maintenance of glycosylated hemoglobin levels <7% to minimize the long-term complications of diabetes, including NPDR and PDR. Similarly, diet and exercise are important adjunctive elements.

Panretinal Photocoagulation

The primary strategy for treatment of PDR is PRP, which involves the widespread placement of laser burns over the entire retina, sparing the central macula (Figure 8-15). The precise mechanism of PRP is not clearly understood. Proposed theories include the destruction of hypoxic retina or the increased diffusion of oxygen from the choroid to supplement the compromised retinal circulation. In both hypotheses, there is a presumed decreased production of vasoproliferative factors, such as VEGF, which leads to inhibition of neovascularization. Application of PRP usually begins as a circular pattern, from approximately 500 μm from the disc and 2 disc diameters from the fovea to avoid the macular center. Full PRP includes the application of laser spots 200 to 500 μm in size, 1 spot size apart, except in areas of neovascularization where the entire area is treated. The procedure is continued peripherally to achieve a total of 1200 to 1600 applications over 2 to 3 sessions. When both macular edema and PDR are present, focal or grid laser treatment is typically performed first for the management of the macular edema. PRP is then performed over 3 to 4 sessions at a later time. In cases that necessitate both procedures concurrently, PRP is applied to the nasal one-third of the retina.

Early support for the use of PRP came from the DRS, a randomized trial evaluating the use of scatter PRP in 1758 patients with PDR in at least one eye or severe NPDR in both eyes. The results showed that PRP reduces the risk of severe visual loss (defined as visual acuity <5/200) by >50%, with the greatest benefit observed in eyes with high-risk characteristics (NVD or vitreous hemorrhage with NVE).[73,74] The ETDRS randomized 3711 patients to early PRP versus deferral, and found that early PRP decreased the risk of high-risk PDR by 50% compared with deferral. Despite the importance of PRP as a therapeutic option, potential complications include loss of peripheral vision, night blindness, color vision change, macular edema, choroidal detachment, glaucoma, and traction retinal detachment.[75]

Vitreoretinal Surgery

When PDR is complicated by severe vitreous hemorrhage or secondary retinal detachment, surgical intervention becomes necessary. When vitrectomy was first introduced in the 1970s, surgical intervention was reserved for long-standing, nonclearing vitreous hemorrhage that lasted for more than 1 year. The Diabetic Retinopathy Vitrectomy Study (DRVS) is a randomized clinical trial that evaluated 616 eyes with recent vitreous hemorrhage to determine whether a role existed for earlier vitrectomy. The results at 2-year follow-up showed improved vision in patients with early vitrectomy (within 6 months) compared with observation, with the benefit maintained at 4-year follow-up in patients with type 1 diabetes.[76-79] With significant improvement in vitreoretinal surgical techniques since the DRVS, including the use of endolaser during surgery, the indications for vitrectomy have widened with improved outcomes.

Traction retinal detachment is another important indication for vitrectomy. Complications from PDR are exacerbated by vitreous traction, resulting in vitreous hemorrhage, traction retinal detachment or schisis, and progressive fibrovascular proliferation. Contraction of the fibrovascular scaffold can lead to retinal breaks and subsequent rhegmatogenous retinal detachment. The presence of chronic retinal detachment contributes to retinal ischemia and significantly increases the risk of further neovascularization.

Currently, primary indications for vitrectomy include PDR with nonclearing vitreous hemorrhage or fibrosis and retinal traction involving or threatening the macula. Based on the DRVS, patients with type 1 diabetes with dense vitreous hemorrhage and severe visual loss in one eye will benefit from early vitrectomy (1 to 6 months after visual loss) rather than waiting >1 year. The study showed no difference in patients with type 2 diabetes, possibly due to the higher rate of diabetic maculopathy in these patients. Although traction retinal detachment not involving the macula may remain stable for years, immediate vitrectomy is indicated when the macula becomes involved. Additional indications for vitrectomy surgery include severe progressive fibrovascular proliferation, epiretinal membrane formation, and persistent diabetic macular edema with associated vitreous traction.

Intravitreal Anti-Angiogenesis Therapy

Given the success of intravitreal anti-VEGF immunotherapy in the treatment of AMD, various clinical trials have evaluated these agents in PDR. Early clinical trials using intravitreal delivery of pegaptanib showed regression of neovascularization.[80] In addition, bevacizumab has been shown to increase the short-term response to PRP in high-risk PDR in select eyes and to be efficacious as an adjuvant treatment to vitrectomy in severe PDR or vitreous hemorrhage.[81] The rationale for such combinatorial therapy is the ability of anti-VEGF agents to reduce active neovascularization and vitreous hemorrhage, allowing PRP or vitrectomy to be performed with fewer complications.

Follow-Up

Of patients with early PDR, 75% will develop high-risk characteristics within 5 years. Therefore, long-term monitoring should include follow-up visits every 2 to 3 months to closely evaluate for disease progression. Once high-risk characteristics are identified, immediate intervention with PRP is warranted. The follow-up interval for patients with high-risk PDR is every 1 to 2 months until the retinopathy has stabilized.

SUMMARY

With the aging population and the rise of obesity and sedentary lifestyle, the incidence of diabetes and its devastating complications will continue to manifest an enlarging burden on our health care and economy. Research has allowed physicians and scientists to better understand the pathogenesis of the ophthalmic complications of diabetes, as well as potential therapeutic options for disrupting the onset or progression of the disease.

Primary prevention of diabetic retinopathy should emphasize glycemic control as well as blood pressure control, as supported by data from the DCCT and UKPDS. Aside from pharmacologic therapy, dietary control and active lifestyle are also important considerations. Although there is also mounting evidence for lipid-lowering agents and anti-platelet therapy, their benefit in diabetic retinopathy remains inconclusive. Additional experimental pharmacological agents are currently under development for both the prevention and treatment of early diabetic retinopathy.

Likewise, secondary interventions in all forms of diabetic retinopathy should continue to emphasize tight control of serum glucose levels and blood pressure. The DRS and ETDRS support the use of PRP in patients with PDR and severe NPDR. Early vitrectomy is reserved primarily for patients with type 1 diabetes with persistent vitreous hemorrhage or hemorrhage preventing other treatments. In patients with diabetic macular edema, focal or grid laser therapy is indicated for reducing the risk of moderate visual loss. Although there is moderate evidence for intravitreal triamcinolone use for diabetic macular edema, further studies are needed to evaluate its long-term safety. Anti-VEGF therapy is another promising new alternative that awaits further clinical evaluation. Future research will be essential to better understand and manage the devastating consequences of diabetic retinopathy.

REFERENCES

1. Centers for Disease Control and Prevention. National diabetes fact sheet: national estimates and general information on diabetes and prediabetes in the United States. Atlanta, GA: US Department of Health and Human Services, Centers for Disease Control and Prevention; 2005.
2. Lightman S, Towler HM. Diabetic retinopathy. *Clin Cornerstone.* 2003;5:12-21.
3. Klein R, Klein BE, Moss SE, Cruickshanks KJ. The Wisconsin Epidemiologic Study of Diabetic Retinopathy: XVII. The 14-year incidence and progression of diabetic retinopathy and associated risk factors in type 1 diabetes. *Ophthalmology.* 1998;105:1801-1815.
4. Harris MI, Klein R, Cowie CC, Rowland M, Byrd-Holt DD. Is the risk of diabetic retinopathy greater in non-Hispanic blacks and Mexican Americans than in non-Hispanic whites with type 2 diabetes? A U.S. population study. *Diabetes Care.* 1998;21:1230-1235.
5. Klein BE, Klein R, Moss SE, Palta M. A cohort study of the relationship of diabetic retinopathy to blood pressure. *Arch Ophthalmol.* 1995;113:601-606.
6. Chew EY, Klein ML, Ferris FL III, et al. Association of elevated serum lipid levels with retinal hard exudate in diabetic retinopathy. Early Treatment Diabetic Retinopathy Study (ETDRS) Report 22. *Arch Ophthalmol.* 1996;114:1079-1084.

7. van Leiden HA, Dekker JM, Moll AC, et al. Blood pressure, lipids, and obesity are associated with retinopathy: the Hoorn study. *Diabetes Care.* 2002;25:1320-1325.

8. Cruickshanks KJ, Ritter LL, Klein R, Moss SE. The association of microalbuminuria with diabetic retinopathy. The Wisconsin Epidemiologic Study of Diabetic Retinopathy. *Ophthalmology.* 1993;100:862-867.

9. Klein BE, Moss SE, Klein R. Effect of pregnancy on progression of diabetic retinopathy. *Diabetes Care.* 1990;13:34-40.

10. Moss SE, Klein R, Klein BE. Association of cigarette smoking with diabetic retinopathy. *Diabetes Care.* 1991;14:119-126.

11. Kriska AM, LaPorte RE, Patrick SL, Kuller LH, Orchard TJ. The association of physical activity and diabetic complications in individuals with insulin-dependent diabetes mellitus: the Epidemiology of Diabetes Complications Study--VII. *J Clin Epidemiol.* 1991;44:1207-1214.

12. The economic impacts of diabetes. International Diabetes Federation Web site. http://www.diabetesatlas.org. Accessed May 2010.

13. Progression of retinopathy with intensive versus conventional treatment in the Diabetes Control and Complications Trial. Diabetes Control and Complications Trial Research Group. *Ophthalmology.* 1995;102:647-661.

14. Intensive blood-glucose control with sulphonylureas or insulin compared with conventional treatment and risk of complications in patients with type 2 diabetes (UKPDS 33). UK Prospective Diabetes Study (UKPDS) Group. *Lancet.* 1998;352:837-853.

15. Zimmer-Galler IE, Zeimer R. Telemedicine in diabetic retinopathy screening. *Int Ophthalmol Clin.* 2009;49:75-86.

16. Aoki N, Dunn K, Fukui T, Beck JR, Schull WJ, Li HK. Cost-effectiveness analysis of telemedicine to evaluate diabetic retinopathy in a prison population. *Diabetes Care.* 2004;27:1095-1101.

17. Wilson C, Horton M, Cavallerano J, Aiello LM. Addition of primary care-based retinal imaging technology to an existing eye care professional referral program increased the rate of surveillance and treatment of diabetic retinopathy. *Diabetes Care.* 2005;28:318-322.

18. Klein R, Palta M, Allen C, Shen G, Han DP, D'Alessio DJ. Incidence of retinopathy and associated risk factors from time of diagnosis of insulin-dependent diabetes. *Arch Ophthalmol.* 1997;115:351-356.

19. The relationship of glycemic exposure (HbA1c) to the risk of development and progression of retinopathy in the diabetes control and complications trial. *Diabetes.* 1995;44:968-983.

20. Kohner EM, Stratton IM, Aldington SJ, Holman RR, Matthews DR. Relationship between the severity of retinopathy and progression to photocoagulation in patients with Type 2 diabetes mellitus in the UKPDS (UKPDS 52). *Diabet Med.* 2001;18:178-184.

21. Frank RN, Keirn RJ, Kennedy A, Frank KW. Galactose-induced retinal capillary basement membrane thickening: prevention by sorbinil. *Invest Ophthalmol Vis Sci.* 1983;24:1519-1524.

22. Gabbay KH. Hyperglycemia, polyol metabolism, and complications of diabetes mellitus. *Annu Rev Med.* 1975;26:521-536.

23. Brownlee M, Vlassara H, Cerami A. Nonenzymatic glycosylation and the pathogenesis of diabetic complications. *Ann Intern Med.* 1984;101:527-537.

24. Wautier JL, Guillausseau PJ. Advanced glycation end products, their receptors and diabetic angiopathy. *Diabetes Metab.* 2001;27:535-542.

25. Giugliano D, Ceriello A, Paolisso G. Oxidative stress and diabetic vascular complications. *Diabetes Care.* 1996;19:257-267.

26. Nishikawa T, Edelstein D, Du XL, et al. Normalizing mitochondrial superoxide production blocks three pathways of hyperglycaemic damage. *Nature.* 2000;404:787-790.

27. Kunisaki M, Bursell SE, Clermont AC, et al. Vitamin E prevents diabetes-induced abnormal retinal blood flow via the diacylglycerol-protein kinase C pathway. *Am J Physiol.* 1995;269:E239-E246.

28. Bursell SE, Clermont AC, Aiello LP, et al. High-dose vitamin E supplementation normalizes retinal blood flow and creatinine clearance in patients with type 1 diabetes. *Diabetes Care.* 1999;22:1245-1251.

29. Aiello LP, Avery RL, Arrigg PG, et al. Vascular endothelial growth factor in ocular fluid of patients with diabetic retinopathy and other retinal disorders. *N Engl J Med.* 1994;331:1480-1487.

30. Wilkinson-Berka JL, Wraight C, Werther G. The role of growth hormone, insulin-like growth factor and somatostatin in diabetic retinopathy. *Curr Med Chem.* 2006;13:3307-3317.

31. Aiello LP, Bursell SE, Clermont A, et al. Vascular endothelial growth factor-induced retinal permeability is mediated by protein kinase C in vivo and suppressed by an orally effective beta-isoform-selective inhibitor. *Diabetes.* 1997;46:1473-1480.

32. Early photocoagulation for diabetic retinopathy. ETDRS report number 9. Early Treatment Diabetic Retinopathy Study Research Group. *Ophthalmology.* 1991;98:766-785.

33. Retinopathy and nephropathy in patients with type 1 diabetes four years after a trial of intensive therapy. The Diabetes Control and Complications Trial/Epidemiology of Diabetes Interventions and Complications Research Group. *N Engl J Med.* 2000;342:381-389.

34. The effect of intensive treatment of diabetes on the development and progression of long-term complications in insulin-dependent diabetes mellitus. The Diabetes Control and Complications Trial Research Group. *N Engl J Med.* 1993;329:977-986.

35. Effect of intensive therapy on the microvascular complications of type 1 diabetes mellitus. *JAMA.* 2002;287:2563-2569.

36. Wang PH, Lau J, Chalmers TC. Meta-analysis of effects of intensive blood-glucose control on late complications of type I diabetes. *Lancet.* 1993;341:1306-1309.

37. Egger M, Davey Smith G, Stettler C, Diem P. Risk of adverse effects of intensified treatment in insulin-dependent diabetes mellitus: a meta-analysis. *Diabet Med.* 1997;14:919-928.

38. Tight blood pressure control and risk of macrovascular and microvascular complications in type 2 diabetes: UKPDS 38. UK Prospective Diabetes Study Group. *BMJ.* 1998;317:703-713.

39. Estacio RO, Jeffers BW, Gifford N, Schrier RW. Effect of blood pressure control on diabetic microvascular complications in patients with hypertension and type 2 diabetes. *Diabetes Care.* 2000;23 Suppl 2:B54-B64.

40. Schrier RW, Estacio RO, Jeffers B. Appropriate Blood Pressure Control in NIDDM (ABCD) Trial. *Diabetologia.* 1996;39:1646-1654.

41. Wilkinson-Berka JL. Angiotensin and diabetic retinopathy. *Int J Biochem Cell Biol.* 2006;38:752-765.

42. Chaturvedi N, Porta M, Klein R, et al. Effect of candesartan on prevention (DIRECT-Prevent 1) and progression (DIRECT-Protect 1) of retinopathy in type 1 diabetes: randomised, placebo-controlled trials. *Lancet.* 2008;372:1394-1402.

43. Sjolie AK, Klein R, Porta M, et al. Effect of candesartan on progression and regression of retinopathy in type 2 diabetes (DIRECT-Protect 2): a randomised placebo-controlled trial. *Lancet.* 2008;372:1385-1393.

44. Matthews DR, Stratton IM, Aldington SJ, Holman RR, Kohner EM. Risks of progression of retinopathy and vision loss related to tight blood pressure control in type 2 diabetes mellitus: UKPDS 69. *Arch Ophthalmol.* 2004;122:1631-1640.

45. Klein R, Sharrett AR, Klein BE, et al. The association of atherosclerosis, vascular risk factors, and retinopathy in adults with diabetes: the atherosclerosis risk in communities study. *Ophthalmology.* 2002;109:1225-1234.

46. Keech AC, Mitchell P, Summanen PA, et al. Effect of fenofibrate on the need for laser treatment for diabetic retinopathy (FIELD study): a randomised controlled trial. *Lancet.* 2007;370:1687-1697.

47. Colhoun HM, Betteridge DJ, Durrington PN, et al. Primary prevention of cardiovascular disease with atorvastatin in type 2 diabetes in the Collaborative Atorvastatin Diabetes Study (CARDS): multicentre randomised placebo-controlled trial. *Lancet.* 2004;364:685-696.

48. Chew EY, Ambrosius WT, Howard LT, et al. Rationale, design, and methods of the Action to Control Cardiovascular Risk in Diabetes Eye Study (ACCORD-EYE). *Am J Cardiol.* 2007;99:103i-111i.

49. Chew EY, Klein ML, Murphy RP, Remaley NA, Ferris FL III. Effects of aspirin on vitreous/preretinal hemorrhage in patients with diabetes mellitus. Early Treatment Diabetic Retinopathy Study report no. 20. *Arch Ophthalmol.* 1995;113:52-55.

50. Effect of aspirin alone and aspirin plus dipyridamole in early diabetic retinopathy. A multicenter randomized controlled clinical trial. The DAMAD Study Group. *Diabetes.* 1989;38:491-498.

51. Sonksen PH, Russell-Jones D, Jones RH. Growth hormone and diabetes mellitus. A review of sixty-three years of medical research and a glimpse into the future? *Horm Res.* 1993;40:68-79.

52. Kirkegaard C, Norgaard K, Snorgaard O, Bek T, Larsen M, Lund-Andersen H. Effect of one year continuous subcutaneous infusion of a somatostatin analogue, octreotide, on early retinopathy, metabolic control and thyroid function in Type I (insulin-dependent) diabetes mellitus. *Acta Endocrinol (Copenh).* 1990;122:766-772.

53. A randomized trial of sorbinil, an aldose reductase inhibitor, in diabetic retinopathy. Sorbinil Retinopathy Trial Research Group. *Arch Ophthalmol.* 1990;108:1234-1244.

54. The effect of ruboxistaurin on visual loss in patients with moderately severe to very severe nonproliferative diabetic retinopathy: initial results of the Protein Kinase C beta Inhibitor Diabetic Retinopathy Study (PKC-DRS) multicenter randomized clinical trial. *Diabetes.* 2005;54:2188-2197.

55. Aiello LP, Davis MD, Girach A, et al. Effect of ruboxistaurin on visual loss in patients with diabetic retinopathy. *Ophthalmology.* 2006;113:2221-2230.

56. Effect of ruboxistaurin in patients with diabetic macular edema: thirty-month results of the randomized PKC-DMES clinical trial. *Arch Ophthalmol.* 2007;125:318-324.

57. Treatment techniques and clinical guidelines for photocoagulation of diabetic macular edema. Early Treatment Diabetic Retinopathy Study Report Number 2. Early Treatment Diabetic Retinopathy Study Research Group. *Ophthalmology.* 1987;94:761-774.

58. Photocoagulation for diabetic macular edema. Early Treatment Diabetic Retinopathy Study report number 1. Early Treatment Diabetic Retinopathy Study research group. *Arch Ophthalmol.* 1985;103:1796-1806.

59. Early Treatment Diabetic Retinopathy Study design and baseline patient characteristics. ETDRS report number 7. *Ophthalmology.* 1991;98:741-756.

60. Stolba U, Binder S, Gruber D, Krebs I, Aggermann T, Neumaier B. Vitrectomy for persistent diffuse diabetic macular edema. *Am J Ophthalmol.* 2005;140:295-301.

61. Yanyali A, Nohutcu AF, Horozoglu F, Celik E. Modified grid laser photocoagulation versus pars plana vitrectomy with internal limiting membrane removal in diabetic macular edema. *Am J Ophthalmol.* 2005;139:795-801.

62. Thomas D, Bunce C, Moorman C, Laidlaw DA. A randomised controlled feasibility trial of vitrectomy versus laser for diabetic macular oedema. *Br J Ophthalmol.* 2005;89:81-86.

63. Gillies MC, Sutter FK, Simpson JM, Larsson J, Ali H, Zhu M. Intravitreal triamcinolone for refractory diabetic macular edema: two-year results of a double-masked, placebo-controlled, randomized clinical trial. *Ophthalmology.* 2006;113:1533-1538.

64. A randomized trial comparing intravitreal triamcinolone acetonide and focal/grid photocoagulation for diabetic macular edema. *Ophthalmology.* 2008;115:1447-1449, 1449.e1-e10.

65. Grover D, Li TJ, Chong CC. Intravitreal steroids for macular edema in diabetes. *Cochrane Database Syst Rev.* 2008:CD005656.

66. Cunningham ET Jr, Adamis AP, Altaweel M, et al. A phase II randomized double-masked trial of pegaptanib, an anti-vascular endothelial growth factor aptamer, for diabetic macular edema. *Ophthalmology.* 2005;112:1747-1757.

67. Shimura M, Nakazawa T, Yasuda K, et al. Comparative therapy evaluation of intravitreal bevacizumab and triamcinolone acetonide on persistent diffuse diabetic macular edema. *Am J Ophthalmol.* 2008;145:854-861.

68. The READ-2 study: ranibizumab for edema of the macula in diabetes. Clinical Trials Web site. http://clinicaltrials.gov. Accessed November 2010.

69. Safety and efficacy of ranibizumab in diabetic macular edema with center involvement (RESOLVE). Clinical Trials Web site. http://clinicaltrials.gov. Accessed November 2010.

70. Scott IU, Edwards AR, Beck RW, et al. A phase II randomized clinical trial of intravitreal bevacizumab for diabetic macular edema. *Ophthalmology.* 2007;114:1860-1867.

71. DME And VEGF Trap-Eye: INvestigation of Clinical Impact (DA VINCI). Clinical Trials Web site. http://clinicaltrials.gov. Accessed November 7, 2008.

72. Preferred Practice Patterns Committee RP. *Diabetic Retinopathy.* San Francisco, CA: American Academy of Ophthalmology; 2003.

73. Photocoagulation treatment of proliferative diabetic retinopathy: the second report of diabetic retinopathy study findings. *Ophthalmology.* 1978;85:82-106.

74. Photocoagulation treatment of proliferative diabetic retinopathy. Clinical application of Diabetic Retinopathy Study (DRS) findings, DRS Report Number 8. The Diabetic Retinopathy Study Research Group. *Ophthalmology.* 1981;88:583-600.

75. Aiello LM. Perspectives on diabetic retinopathy. *Am J Ophthalmol.* 2003;136:122-135.

76. Early vitrectomy for severe vitreous hemorrhage in diabetic retinopathy. Two-year results of a randomized trial. Diabetic Retinopathy Vitrectomy Study report 2. The Diabetic Retinopathy Vitrectomy Study Research Group. *Arch Ophthalmol.* 1985;103:1644-1652.

77. Early vitrectomy for severe vitreous hemorrhage in diabetic retinopathy. Four-year results of a randomized trial: Diabetic Retinopathy Vitrectomy Study Report 5. *Arch Ophthalmol.* 1990;108:958-964.

78. Early vitrectomy for severe proliferative diabetic retinopathy in eyes with useful vision. Results of a randomized trial--Diabetic Retinopathy Vitrectomy Study Report 3. The Diabetic Retinopathy Vitrectomy Study Research Group. *Ophthalmology.* 1988;95:1307-1320.

79. Early vitrectomy for severe proliferative diabetic retinopathy in eyes with useful vision. Clinical application of results of a randomized trial--Diabetic Retinopathy Vitrectomy Study Report 4. The Diabetic Retinopathy Vitrectomy Study Research Group. *Ophthalmology.* 1988;95:1321-1334.

80. Adamis AP, Altaweel M, Bressler NM, et al. Changes in retinal neovascularization after pegaptanib (Macugen) therapy in diabetic individuals. *Ophthalmology.* 2006;113:23-28.

81. Arevalo JF, Garcia-Amaris RA. Intravitreal bevacizumab for diabetic retinopathy. *Curr Diabetes Rev.* 2009;5:39-46.

9

Perspectives in Ocular Telemedicine Imaging for Diabetes Mellitus

Paolo S. Silva, MD; Lloyd M. Aiello, MD; Lloyd Paul Aiello, MD, PhD; Dorothy Tolls, OD; and Jerry D. Cavallerano, OD, PhD

The prevalence of retinal imaging programs, using a store and forward approach with the transmission of digital retinal images for grading to assess for the presence and/or severity of diabetic retinopathy, has increased significantly in the past decade. Such programs have been established in both highly industrialized nations and developing countries, but programs have varied widely in goals and approach, providing significantly varying levels of diabetes eye care to the intended target population. Often inappropriately described as "screening" for diabetic retinopathy, telemedicine for diabetic retinopathy has become increasingly common across all types of health care systems that include federally funded health care agencies in the United States; national health care systems in Europe, Asia, and Australia; private health care companies; and commercial business enterprises. This chapter provides a general overview of telemedicine for diabetic retinopathy and describes the benefits and challenges associated with establishing such programs. Extensive reviews of the different ocular telemedicine programs for diabetic retinopathy[1,2] and the comprehensive approach to total diabetes care[3-5] may serve as additional references to supplement this chapter.

THE NECESSITY OF TELEMEDICINE FOR DIABETIC RETINOPATHY

The continuously increasing prevalence of diabetes worldwide and the relative shortage of qualified eye care professionals to provide highly effective, evidenced-based treatments for diabetic retinopathy suggest that the most practical method to care for all persons with diabetes in the twenty-first century is to utilize an effective telemedicine program.

THE PROBLEM

By the year 2030, it is estimated that 439 million people worldwide will have diabetes mellitus.[6] Reducing the risks of microvascular and macrovascular complications of diabetes is essential to maintaining health and the quality of life of people with diabetes. Although present recommendations and treatment for

Espaillat A.
Diabetic Eye Disease: A Comprehensive Review (pp. 91-100)
© 2012 SLACK Incorporated

diabetic retinal complications are extremely effective, the access to appropriate eye care remains a significant barrier, leading to undiagnosed advanced disease and resulting in visual loss accompanied by a staggering loss of human and economic resources. In 2009, the direct and indirect diabetes-related health expenditure in the United States alone was $113 billion, and if no interventions are implemented, at the current rate it is expected to more than triple by 2034.[7]

Given this increased incidence and prevalence of diabetes and the significant improvements in medical care leading to increased life expectancy of people with diabetes, it is expected that the rate of diabetic eye complications will continue to rise. Population-based studies have shown that after 15 years of diabetes, the development of overt diabetic retinopathy occurs in 96% of people with type 1 diabetes[8] and in >60% of people with type 2 diabetes.[9] Furthermore, despite advances in eye care, diabetic retinopathy remains the leading cause of new-onset adult blindness in working-age adults in the United States and other developed nations. Sight-threatening changes from diabetic retinopathy are readily diagnosed with ophthalmic examination and can be treatable with timely intervention, but more than one-third of patients in the United States do not obtain regular eye care due to a variety of factors.[10] This lack of appropriate eye care is even more pronounced in developing countries and may be the result of a combination of factors such as the asymptomatic nature of the early stages of diabetic retinopathy; patient and provider unawareness of potential visual complications; and no or limited access brought about by socioeconomic, psychosocial, or cultural barriers that hinder eye care delivery.

Currently, the overall 25-year incidence of visual impairment (visual acuity of 20/40 or worse) is 13% and the incidence of severe visual impairment (20/200 or worse) is 3% among patients with type 1 diabetes in the United States. According to a recent Wisconsin Epidemiologic Study of Diabetic Retinopathy (WESDR) report, cataracts, more severe baseline diabetic retinopathy, higher hemoglobin A1c (HbA1c), hypertension, and smoking are strongly associated with risk for visual impairment among patients with diabetes.[11]

Innovative methods of eye care delivery are needed to address the rise in the prevalence of diabetes and its complications. Poor health maintenance and lack of access to care due to a variety of personal, geographical, and socioeconomic reasons increase the risk of diabetes complications. Interventions to prevent visual loss and preserve vision are most effective during the early stages of diabetic retinopathy when the majority of patients are unaware of problems and the disease is largely asymptomatic. This asymptomatic nature of the disease emphasizes the importance of retinal examinations to detect and evaluate disease severity and identify patients at risk for vision loss. To provide the minimum requirement of an annual eye examination to each of the 439 million people expected to have diabetes by 2030, 2.4 million eyes will need to be examined every day with the number continuously rising. The capability to meet this global burden remains unmet and continues to be a significant public health concern that stresses the health care system. An effective health care model of diabetes eye care that can cope with the growing need and provide the greatest benefit for people with diabetes should be established.

The Solution

Evidence-Based Care

To preserve vision and prevent vision loss from diabetes, effective evidence-based care must be available to all persons with diabetes and novel, more effective treatments and preventive measures that will eventually lead to a definitive cure must be developed. This level of care should be made available to all patients and potentially accessible wherever the patient is located. Evidence-based care has demonstrated that many of the changes in diabetic retinopathy that lead to vision loss are preventable and/or treatable.

More than 40 years of clinical trials have established the current evidence-based care for diabetic retinopathy (Table 9-1). The Diabetic Retinopathy Study (DRS),[12] Early Treatment of Diabetic Retinopathy Study (ETDRS),[13-15] Diabetes Control and Complications Trail (DCCT),[16] Epidemiology of Diabetes Interventions and Complications (EDIC),[17,18] United Kingdom Prospective Diabetes Study (UKPDS),[19,20] and Diabetic Retinopathy Clinical Research Network (DRCR. net)[21,22] have demonstrated the effectiveness of laser surgery in treating diabetic retinopathy and diabetic macular edema; the value of intensive and consistent glycemic control; the importance of controlling comorbidities such as hypertension, hypercholesterolemia, dyslipidemia, anemia, and renal disease; and the role of novel therapies such as intravitreal vascular endothelial cell growth factor (VEGF) inhibitors and intravitreal steroids. Advances in diabetes care, including improved methods of continuously monitoring and controlling blood glucose levels, provide the opportunity to significantly lower glycosylated HbA1C levels while reducing the risk of hyperglycemia and hypoglycemia. Most importantly, early detection, preventive care, and treatment of diabetic eye disease lead to improved long-term visual outcomes.

Table 9-1. Evidence-Based Diabetic Retinopathy Care

Study	Major Findings
Diabetic Retinopathy Study (DRS)[12]	Scatter photocoagulation reduced the risk of severe vision loss by >50% for eyes with high-risk PDR
Early Treatment Diabetic Retinopathy Study (ETDRS)[13-15]	Focal laser photocoagulation for clinically significant macular edema reduced the risk of moderate vision loss by >50% and increased the chance of a small improvement in visual acuity. Both early scatter laser photocoagulation and deferral until high-risk retinopathy developed had low rates of severe visual loss (5-year rates in deferral subgroups 2% to 10%; in early photocoagulation groups, 2% to 6%). The benefit of early treatment was more pronounced in type 2 diabetes and type 1 diabetes of long duration. 650 mg of aspirin had no effect on progression of retinopathy, frequency of vitreous hemorrhage, or cataract development.
Diabetes Control and Complications Trial (DCCT)[16]/ Epidemiology of Diabetes Intervention and Complications (EDIC)[17,18]	Intensive blood glucose control for type 1 diabetes Primary prevention: • 27% reduction in development of diabetic retinopathy • 78% reduction in 3-step progression of diabetic retinopathy Secondary intervention: • 54% reduction in 3-step progression of diabetic retinopathy • 47% reduction in PDR and severe NPDR • 56% reduction in photocoagulation • 23% reduction in macular edema
United Kingdom Prospective Diabetes Study (UKPDS)[19,20]	Intensive blood glucose control for type 1 diabetes—Effects of intensive therapy persist for at least 10 years after differences in glycemia between the original intensive and conventional therapy groups. • 29% reduction in need for laser • 17% reduction in 2-step progression of diabetic retinopathy • 24% reduction in need for cataract extraction • 23% reduction in vitreous hemorrhage • 16% reduction in legal blindness • Continued benefit after 10 years despite convergence of HbA1C levels after 1 year

PDR = proliferative diabetic retinopathy, NPDR = nonproliferative diabetic retinopathy

Telemedicine

Because diabetes mellitus is a complex chronic disease that requires lifelong care, telemedicine provides the means for global access, assessment, diagnosis and care, and evidence-based treatment of all patients with diabetes mellitus and diabetic retinopathy across geographic, socioeconomic, and cultural barriers.

The American Telemedicine Association (ATA) clearly elucidates the meaning and characteristics of telemedicine[23]:

> [Telemedicine is] the use of medical information exchanged from one site to another via electronic communications to improve patients' health status. Closely associated with telemedicine is the term "telehealth," which is often used to encompass a broader definition of remote health care that does not always involve clinical services. Videoconferencing, transmission of still images, e-health including patient portals, remote monitoring of vital signs, continuing medical education, and nursing call centers are all considered part of telemedicine and telehealth.
>
> Telemedicine is not a separate medical specialty. Products and services related to telemedicine are often part of a larger investment by health care institutions in either information technology or the delivery of clinical care. Even in the reimbursement fee structure, there is usually no distinction made between services provided on site and those provided through telemedicine and often no separate coding required for billing of remote services.

In the most basic sense, telemedicine programs may simply consist of the acquisition of patient health information such as a blood glucose measurement or of a set of retinal images to determine the presence or severity level of diabetic retinopathy to provide triage recommendations for referral to tertiary medical centers. This basic model of telemedicine provides some public health benefit but places an undue burden on an already overwhelmed acute care medical system. The experience at the Veterans Affairs Healthcare System in Togus, ME, illustrates this problem; following deployment of a telemedicine program at the facility, a large increase in eye care referrals occurred that could not be met by the medical center in a timely fashion. The population was predominantly older males with type 2 diabetes, and 74.5% of patients had no diabetic retinopathy or mild nonproliferative diabetic retinopathy (NPDR) as their most severe ocular finding; conversely, 25.5% of patients had at least one eye with moderate NPDR or worse. Additionally, 58.7% of patients with no or mild diabetic retinopathy had at least one nondiabetic ocular finding of a severity that necessitated referral, resulting in a large population identified requiring eye care.[24] Although the telemedicine program provided the critical function of detecting significant retinopathy and other retinal disorders, thus reducing the number of patients who might otherwise be inappropriately deferred based solely on retinopathy findings, the increased access to patients resulted in an increased number of eye care referrals. A telemedicine program designed to offer ongoing care for patients with no or mild disease, thereby deferring an in-person examination, would allow resources to be directed to patients with more significant findings, thereby relieving an undue burden to the health care system.

Telemedicine programs for diabetic retinopathy are often mislabeled as "screening programs." Traditionally, the concept of "screening" has been applied to laboratory tests, physical examination, or radiologic tests performed on asymptomatic patients without known disease to uncover subclinical disease.[25] Once the disease has been identified and medical care and treatment are undertaken, this process now becomes the practice of medicine—telemedicine. Telemedicine for diabetic retinopathy deals with patients who have been diagnosed with diabetes; whether retinopathy is clinically evident or not, these patients require evidence-based care and comprehensive diabetes management, and this level of care no longer falls within the accepted concept of screening. Furthermore, telemedicine diabetes eye care programs have the potential to enhance the practice of medicine by utilizing information technology to integrate results from multiple diagnostic evaluations and patient health information within a single interactive electronic medical/health record, providing an appropriate treatment plan and follow-up during the life of the patient across geographic and socioeconomic barriers.

Innovative and novel telemedicine programs can be designed, tested, and deployed to meet the need of diabetes eye care. Current retinal imaging systems can accurately identify and evaluate diabetic retinopathy severity, which have been shown to be comparable to the gold standard 7-field ETDRS photography or to an in-person retinal examination for diabetic retinopathy.[26] Combining retinal image acquisition with a comprehensive electronic medical record, an accurate and comprehensive assessment of a patient's risk for the development or progression of diabetic retinopathy can be provided. Such programs will allow for timely and appropriate management recommendations for patients with diabetic retinopathy to be given through telemedicine. Additionally, comprehensive patient health information that includes photographic documentation of retinal disease severity can be utilized in epidemiologic research and potentially lead to the identification of retinal lesions that may be predictive or protective of progressive retinopathy in the future.

Preliminary results from a pilot program that integrates epidemiologic research and the prospective evaluation for retinal biomarkers are promising. A remote site pediatric diabetes eye care program was established in 2006 at the Pediatric Endocrine Clinic at the Hospital de Niños JM de los Rios in Caracas, Venezuela, to provide access to retinal evaluations and provide management recommendations. With the use of a telemedicine diabetes eye care program, more than 311 patients have received diabetes eye care and 134 patients received follow-up retinal imaging, with systematic gathering of pertinent data including patient demographics and medical and diabetes history, the results of which have influenced diabetes care practice patterns within the hospital. Retinal images are currently being prospectively evaluated for retinal vascular changes in the form of capillary dilation, shunting, and drop-out in the midperiphery of the retina, which are presumed to be closely correlated with the development of overt diabetic retinopathy.[27]

Scientific Validation

Although telemedicine for diabetic retinopathy has the potential to provide evidence-based diabetic eye care that is fully integrated with total diabetes care, such programs must be clearly defined and validated to ensure the level of care provided. Recognizing the importance of clearly defined expectations and the need to provide evidence-based care through telemedicine programs, the ATA published *Telehealth Practice Recommendations for Diabetic Retinopathy.*[28] Like the ETDRS 30-degree stereo 7-standard fields, color 35-mm slides (ETDRS photographs) are an accepted standard for evaluating diabetic retinopathy, the guidelines accepted ETDRS photographs as the criteria to

Table 9-2. Clinical Categories of Validation

Category 1	Separates patients into 2 categories: (1) those who have no or very mild NPDR and (2) those with levels more severe than mild NPDR.
Category 2	Indicates a system can accurately determine whether sight-threatening diabetic retinopathy (as evidenced by any level of diabetic macular edema, severe or worse levels of NPDR, or PDR) are present or not present.
Category 3	Indicates a system can identify ETDRS defined levels of NPDR (mild, moderate, or severe), PDR (non–high-risk or high-risk), and diabetic macular edema with accuracy sufficient to determine appropriate follow-up and treatment strategies.
Category 4	Indicates a system matches or exceeds the ability of ETDRS photographs to identify lesions of diabetic retinopathy to determine levels of diabetic retinopathy and diabetic macular edema.

NPDR = nonproliferative diabetic retinopathy, PDR = proliferative diabetic retinopathy, ETDRS = Early Treatment Diabetic Retinopathy Study

assess the accuracy of a telemedicine system for diabetic retinopathy.[29] The ATA guidelines recommend that telehealth programs for diabetic retinopathy should compare favorably with ETDRS photographs as reflected in kappa values for agreement of diagnosis, false positive and false negative readings, positive predictive value, negative predictive value, and sensitivity and specificity of diagnosing levels of retinopathy and macular edema. The inability to obtain or read images is considered a positive finding for disease. There are standards other than ETDRS photographs, however. Telemedicine programs should clarify the standards used for validation and relevant data sets used for comparison if ETDRS photographs are not used. Telemedicine programs for diabetic retinopathy should clearly define their goals and performance in relationship to accepted clinical standards. The Telehealth Practice Recommendations for Diabetic Retinopathy prepared by the ATA clearly delineate performance standards for clinical, technical, and administrative elements of ocular telemedicine for diabetic retinopathy.

Four clinical categories of assessment are identified in the ATA Practice Recommendations (Table 9-2). Category 1 validation separates patients into 2 categories: those who have no or virtually no diabetic retinopathy present (ETDRS level 20 or below) versus those who have diabetic retinopathy apparently present.[29] Functionally, this level of validation identifies patients who have no or minimal diabetic retinopathy and those who have more than minimal diabetic retinopathy. Category 2 validation allows identification of patients who do not have sight-threatening diabetic retinopathy and those who have potentially sight-threatening diabetic retinopathy. This level of validation indicates the program accurately determines whether sight-threatening diabetic retinopathy is present, as evidenced by any level of macular edema, severe or worse levels of NPDR (ETDRS level 53 or worse), or proliferative diabetic retinopathy (PDR). Category 3 validation indicates a system can identify ETDRS-defined levels of NPDR (mild, moderate, or severe), PDR (non–high-risk, high-risk), and diabetic macular edema with accuracy sufficient to determine appropriate follow-up and treatment strategies. This level of validation allows patient management to match clinical recommendations based on clinical retinal examination through dilated pupils. Category 4 validation indicates that a system matches or exceeds the ability of ETDRS photographs to identify all of the specific lesions of diabetic retinopathy, which leads to the determination of "levels of diabetic retinopathy" and "diabetic macular edema." Functionally, category 4 validation indicates that a program can replace ETDRS photographs in any clinical or research program.

Clinical validation of a program or imaging modality is not defined solely by the number and composition of retinal fields, but goes beyond retinal images and is based on the clinical protocol by which images are evaluated and the level of treatment recommendations that are provided to patients. Each program and imaging modality should undergo rigorous scientific validation against the standard of care, and findings in one system and/or program should not be extrapolated to similar but invalidated systems and/or programs.

Peer-reviewed validation studies on telemedicine programs for diabetic retinopathy have been extensively reported in the literature and have been summarized in previous reviews.[1] Validation studies should be specific to each program and the goals it wishes to attain. Comparison must be performed with the standard of care,[26] against a clinical examination,[30] and as a substitute for clinical examination.[31]

Table 9-3. Technical Considerations

Image Acquisition	Image data set must use DICOM standards and include DICOM image information in the image headers
Compression	Reversible and irreversible compression should undergo clinical validation for diagnostic accuracy
Data Communication/ Transfer	Transmission should have no loss of clinically significant information, should be DICOM compliant and accompanied by a current DICOM conformance statement, and should include error-checking capabilities
Archiving and Retrieval	Storage should comply with facility, state, and federal regulations for medical record retention and be equivalent to policies for protection of hard copy storage media to preserve imaging records
Security	All systems must be HIPAA compliant
Reliability and Redundancy	Images should be retained as part of the patient's medical record to meet clinical needs of facility and medical staff
Documentation	Reports of findings should be compliant with DICOM standard for structured reports

DICOM = Digital Imaging and Communications in Medicine, HIPAA = Health Insurance Portability and Accountability Act

Table 9-4. Operational and Business Elements

Operational	• Integrate ocular telehealth with primary care of diabetes consistent with accepted standards • Preserve doctor-patient relationship, ensure quality of images and image evaluation, and ensure adherence to recommendations • Ensure appropriate communication and qualifications of personnel • Provide appropriate system and data maintenance, security, integrity, and recovery
Legal/ Regulatory	• Assure appropriate licensure and accreditation of all personnel • Preserve HIPAA compliance for data privacy, integrity, security, retrieval, and patient consent • Provide liability coverage through appropriate risk management and insurance • Obtain patient consent emphasizing the difference between comprehensive eye examination and telehealth program, and the benefits and risks of program • Establish quality management, standardized training, ongoing evaluation, continuing education, and performance improvement
Financial	• Establish program sustainability through a well-developed business plan

Technology considerations for any telemedicine program are summarized in Table 9-3 and include recommendations in the following areas: image acquisition and analysis, data compression and transfer, display capabilities, archiving and retrieval, security, reliability and redundancy, and documentation and the recommendations. Specifically, any imaging acquisition system used should be Digital Imaging and Communications in Medicine (DICOM) standard compliance,[32] and the patient health information record system should comply with Health Insurance Portability and Accountability Act (HIPAA)[33] regulations.

Operational and business recommendations are summarized in Table 9-4 and address key aspects of the program, which include safety and effectiveness of system deployment, ethics of doctor-patient relationship, jurisdictional and community standards, qualifications of imagers and readers, supervisory personnel, system maintenance, data security and disaster recovery, cross-border provider licensure and credentialing, quality assurance and control, financial liabilities, and operational sustainability.

General Approaches of Telemedicine Programs for Diabetic Retinopathy

The scope and intent of ocular telemedicine for diabetes vary significantly and have traditionally been tailored to address the needs of the intended population, but the increased prevalence of diabetes is not an isolated problem and should be addressed on a global scale. Ideally, ocular telemedicine programs for diabetes should have the capability for integration within a diverse spectrum of settings including primary care settings, sequestered populations such as in prison or penal institutions, remote areas with limited health care facilities, underserved populations, and hospital-based or tertiary care facilities. Current programs in the United States are operating in the Indian Health Service, US Department of Defense, and US Veterans Administration. Academic institutions and private corporations also have developed programs. Canada, England, and many European and Asian countries have utilized telemedicine for diabetic retinopathy. Significant reviews on the different ocular telemedicine programs have been published,[1,2] and only a general approach is discussed in succeeding paragraphs.

Ocular telemedicine for diabetic retinopathy can function in a variety of roles. Telemedicine programs can provide care where access to eye care is limited due to geographic or socioeconomic barriers. Even within established health care settings, telemedicine may overcome patient resistance to eye examination through the use of nonmydriatic imaging and by locating imaging services at the point of service for other health care needs, such as primary care provider visits or other health care encounters. In this sense, ocular telemedicine provides access to eye care, with an opportunity to incorporate patient education in addition to the benefits of regular eye examination for diabetic retinopathy.

Planned, well-designed telemedicine programs using retinal imaging and reporting diagnosis and treatment plans can also serve as alternative methods to provide routine diabetic eye care. Such programs can provide careful follow-up and allow timely treatment to prevent onset of diabetic retinopathy and to monitor for the onset or progression of diabetic retinopathy in remote and established locations. Telemedicine may substitute for periodic clinical retinal examination during pregnancy, for persons initiating intensive glucose control, and for persons with less than severe levels of diabetic retinopathy. ATA category 3 and 4 ocular telemedicine programs allow for photographic documentation of retinal lesions and use a standard protocol for retinal evaluation, which can be used as a means to identify individuals who may be eligible for and benefit from participation in clinical trials and, if rigorously validated, may serve as a means to assess diabetic retinopathy severity longitudinally in participants of clinical trials.[34,35]

A distinct advantage of ocular telemedicine for diabetic retinopathy is directly related to its inherent use of information technology, which easily allows the full integration of diabetes eye care into a comprehensive diabetes care program for each individual. Ocular telemedicine at the point of care in a primary care, endocrine office or any other health care setting allows a virtually immediate assessment of diabetic retinopathy that may significantly impact the patient's medical care. This assessment provides eye care recommendations and the appropriate interval for eye care follow-up for the patient, and the identified level of eye disease may influence medical therapeutic approaches and management of existing comorbidities.

Challenges of Establishing an Ocular Telemedicine Program

Telemedicine programs face multiple inherent challenges. Technological advances are rapid and may render the technology of any system obsolete within 3 to 5 years. Upgrades may be costly and time consuming, and new components require constant validation and integration with previous medical records. To overcome these obstacles, fiscal and financial strategies should be designed and implemented to ensure that the clinical programs meet the standard of evidence-based care and that information technology is enhanced to meet the telemedicine clinical program needs. The human factors in a telemedicine program, which may introduce errors in encoding and interpretation of patient health information and/or treatment plans, should be minimized to ensure delivery of the standard evidence-based medical care by automating the telemedicine processes, including image acquisition, evaluation, diagnosis, and treatment recommendations. Initially, telemedicine programs may be met with significant resistance and may not fully integrate into an already established model of care. This initial reluctance to adopt a telemedicine program may be due to an inherent resistance to change and misconceptions about the technology and the disease by patients, and more so, by caregivers. It has been repeatedly shown that the adoption of an ocular telemedicine program for diabetic retinopathy has resulted in significant benefits in terms of the reduction of health care expenditure[36,37] and increasing scope of eye care delivery,[38] which should, in theory, ameliorate these concerns.

Several recurring regulatory and legal challenges face telemedicine programs, principally due to the often varying geographic locations and regulatory constraints between the patient and care provider. Attempts on standardization that would limit operational challenges and address these recurring issues have been published by the ATA[28] and are summarized in Table 9-3. Considerations include local and national regulations concerning patient privacy, regulatory mandates, malpractice insurance and liability, licensure and credentialing, and reimbursement from third-party payers. Although still not yet widely accepted, the development of these standards provides the basic framework of establishing a telemedicine program for diabetic retinopathy.

FUTURE EXPECTATIONS

Today, telemedicine diabetes eye care programs are only partially effective in providing varying degrees of benefits. Without appropriate programmatic and technological enhancements, they cannot meet the near-future challenge of caring for the increasing number of persons with diabetes worldwide because of their inability to provide the necessary remote site evaluations, treatments, and careful follow-up. Image acquisition systems will, of necessity, become truly portable, handheld, high-resolution, and high quality. Retinal assessment will move beyond the concept of traditional retinal photographs toward the use of computational algorithms for lesion detection analysis or of other imaging modalities, such as new scanning laser-based imaging systems, that can lead to the identification of very early retinal vascular changes or angiogenic growth factors that may be predictive of the onset and/or progression of diabetic retinopathy. Gradually, other elements of the comprehensive eye examination, such as visual acuity and intraocular pressure measurements, will be included.

By 2030, 439 million patients with diabetes mellitus will require specialized and long-term eye care. Based on the evidence-based standards, 28 eyes per second, 365 days per year every year will require evaluation for level of diabetic retinopathy, treatment, and careful follow-up.[6] This demand will overwhelm the current medical and eye care system. Telemedicine will soon be a mainstay of health care delivery worldwide. Ocular telemedicine for diabetic retinopathy is vital for the eye care and total care of persons with diabetes. The realization of a comprehensive diabetes care program telemedicine network available to virtually each patient on a global scale should be the mission and goal to ensure patients with diabetes an acceptable quality of life until prevention and cure is attained for all.

REFERENCES

1. Silva PS, Cavallerano JD, Aiello LM. Ocular telehealth initiatives in diabetic retinopathy. *Curr Diab Rep*. 2009;9:265-271.
2. Silva PS, Cavallerano JD, Aiello LM, Aiello LP. Telemedicine and diabetic retinopathy: moving beyond retinal screening. *Arch Ophthalmol*. 2011;129:236-242.
3. Silva PS, Cavallerano JD, Sun JK, Aiello LM, Aiello LP. Effect of systemic on onset and progression of diabetic retinopathy. *Nat Rev Endocrinol*. 2010;6:494-508.
4. Fonda SJ, Bursell SE, Lewis DG, Garren J, Hock K, Cavallerano J. The relationship of a diabetes telehealth eye care program to standard eye care and change in diabetes health outcomes. *Telemed J E Health*. 2007;13:635-644.
5. Fonda SJ, Paulsen CA, Perkins J, Kedziora RJ, Rodbard D, Bursell SE. Usability test of an internet-based informatics tool for diabetes care providers: the comprehensive diabetes management program. *Diabetes Technol Ther*. 2008;10:16-24.
6. Shaw JE, Sicree RA, Zimmet PZ. Global estimates of the prevalence of diabetes for 2010 and 2030. *Diabetes Res Clin Pract*. 2010;87:4-14.
7. Huang ES, Basu A, O'Grady M, Capretta JC. Projecting the future diabetes population size and related costs for the U.S. *Diabetes Care*. 2009;32:2225-2229.
8. Klein R, Klein BE, Moss SE, Davis MD, DeMets DL. The Wisconsin Epidemiologic Study of Diabetic Retinopathy. II. Prevalence and risk of diabetic retinopathy when age at diagnosis is less than 30 years. *Arch Ophthalmol*. 1984;102:520-526.
9. Klein R, Klein BE, Moss SE, Davis MD, DeMets DL. The Wisconsin Epidemiologic Study of Diabetic Retinopathy. III. Prevalence and risk of diabetic retinopathy when age at diagnosis is 30 or more years. *Arch Ophthalmol*. 1984;102:527-532.
10. Schoenfeld ER, Greene JM, Wu SY, Leske MC. Patterns of adherence to diabetes vision care guidelines: baseline findings from the Diabetic Retinopathy Awareness Program. *Ophthalmology*. 2001;108:563-571.
11. Klein R, Lee KE, Gangnon RE, Klein BE. The 25-year incidence of visual impairment in type 1 diabetes mellitus. The Wisconsin Epidemiologic Study of Diabetic Retinopathy. *Ophthalmology*. 2010;117:63-70.
12. Photocoagulation treatment of proliferative diabetic retinopathy. Clinical application of Diabetic Retinopathy Study (DRS) findings, DRS Report Number 8. The Diabetic Retinopathy Study Research Group. *Ophthalmology*. 1981;88:583-600.
13. Photocoagulation for diabetic macular edema. Early Treatment Diabetic Retinopathy Study report number 1. Early Treatment Diabetic Retinopathy Study research group. *Arch Ophthalmol*. 1985;103:1796-1806.
14. Early photocoagulation for diabetic retinopathy. ETDRS report number 9. Early Treatment Diabetic Retinopathy Study Research Group. *Ophthalmology*. 1991;98:766-785.
15. Effects of aspirin treatment on diabetic retinopathy. ETDRS report number 8. Early Treatment Diabetic Retinopathy Study Research Group. *Ophthalmology*. 1991;98:757-765.
16. The effect of intensive treatment of diabetes on the development and progression of long-term complications in insulin-dependent diabetes mellitus. The Diabetes Control and Complications Trial Research Group. *N Engl J Med*. 1993;329:977-986.
17. Sustained effect of intensive treatment of type 1 diabetes mellitus on development and progression of diabetic nephropathy: the Epidemiology of Diabetes Interventions and Complications (EDIC) study. *JAMA*. 2003;290:2159-2167.
18. White NH, Sun W, Cleary PA, et al. Prolonged effect of intensive therapy on the risk of retinopathy complications in patients with type 1 diabetes mellitus: 10 years after the Diabetes Control and Complications Trial. *Arch Ophthalmol*. 2008;126:1707-1715.

19. Intensive blood-glucose control with sulphonylureas or insulin compared with conventional treatment and risk of complications in patients with type 2 diabetes (UKPDS 33). UK Prospective Diabetes Study (UKPDS) Group. *Lancet*. 1998;352:837-853.

20. Holman RR, Paul SK, Bethel MA, Matthews DR, Neil HA. 10-year follow-up of intensive glucose control in type 2 diabetes. *N Engl J Med*. 2008;359:1577-1589.

21. Elman MJ, Aiello LP, Beck RW, et al; Diabetic Retinopathy Clinical Research Network. Randomized trial evaluating ranibizumab plus prompt or deferred laser or triamcinolone plus prompt laser for diabetic macular edema. *Ophthalmology*. 2010;117:1064-1077.e35.

22. Diabetic Retinopathy Clinical Research Network. A randomized trial comparing intravitreal triamcinolone acetonide and focal/grid photocoagulation for diabetic macular edema. *Ophthalmology*. 2008;115:1447-1449, 1449.e1-e10.

23. American Telemedicine Association. Telemedicine defined. American Telemed Association Web site. http://www.americantelemed.org/i4a/pages/index.cfm?pageid=3333. Accessed November 2011.

24. Cavallerano AA, Cavallerano JD, Katalinic P, et al. A telemedicine program for diabetic retinopathy in a Veterans Affairs Medical Center–the Joslin Vision Network Eye Health Care Model. *Am J Ophthalmol*. 2005;139:597-604.

25. Nielsen C, Lang RS. Principles of screening. *Med Clin North Am*. 1999;83:1323-1337.

26. Bursell SE, Cavallerano JD, Cavallerano AA, et al. Stereo non-mydriatic digital-video color retinal imaging compared with Early Treatment Diabetic Retinopathy Study seven standard field 35-mm stereo color photos for determining level of diabetic retinopathy. *Ophthalmology*. 2001;108:572-585.

27. Silva PS, Hock K, Grossmann MM, Sun JK, Cavallerano JD, Aiello LM. Joslin Vision Network: Pediatric Diabetes Ocular Telemedicine Program. *Telemed J E Health*. 2009;15:719.

28. Cavallerano J, Lawrence MG, Zimmer-Galler I, et al. Telehealth practice recommendations for diabetic retinopathy. *Telemed J E Health*. 2004;10:469-482.

29. Grading diabetic retinopathy from stereoscopic color fundus photographs--an extension of the modified Airlie House classification. ETDRS report number 10. Early Treatment Diabetic Retinopathy Study Research Group. *Ophthalmology*. 1991;98:786-806.

30. Cavallerano AA, Cavallerano JD, Katalinic P, Tolson AM, Aiello LP, Aiello LM. Use of Joslin Vision Network digital-video nonmydriatic retinal imaging to assess diabetic retinopathy in a clinical program. *Retina*. 2003;23:215-223.

31. Cavallerano JD, Cavallerano JD, Katalinic P, et al. Nonmydriatic digital imaging alternative for annual retinal examination in persons with previously documented no or mild diabetic retinopathy. *Am J Ophthalmol*. 2005;140:667-673.

32. Bidgood WD Jr, Horii SC. Introduction to the ACR-NEMA DICOM standard. *Radiographics*. 1992;12:345-355.

33. Office of the National Coordinator for Health Information Technology, Department of Health and Human Services. Health information technology: initial set of standards, implementation specifications, and certification criteria for electronic health record technology. Interim final rule. *Fed Regist*. 2010;75:2013-2047.

34. Last D, Alsop DC, Abduljalil AM, et al. Global and regional effects of type 2 diabetes on brain tissue volumes and cerebral vasoreactivity. *Diabetes Care*. 2007;30:1193-1199.

35. Novak V, Last D, Alsop DC, et al. Cerebral blood flow velocity and periventricular white matter hyperintensities in type 2 diabetes. *Diabetes Care*. 2006;29:1529-1534.

36. Jones S, Edwards RT. Diabetic retinopathy screening: a systematic review of the economic evidence. *Diabet Med*. 2010;27:249-256.

37. Whited JD, Datta SK, Aiello LM, et al. A modeled economic analysis of a digital tele-ophthalmology system as used by three federal health care agencies for detecting proliferative diabetic retinopathy. *Telemed J E Health*. 2005;11:641-651.

38. Conlin PR, Fisch BM, Orcutt JC, Hetrick BJ, Darkins AW. Framework for a national teleretinal imaging program to screen for diabetic retinopathy in Veterans Health Administration patients. *J Rehabil Res Dev*. 2006;43:741-748.

Financial Disclosures

Dr. Lloyd M. Aiello has no financial or proprietary interest in the materials presented herein.

Dr. Lloyd Paul Aiello has no financial or proprietary interest in the materials presented herein.

Dr. Larissa Camejo is a consultant for Allergan and Alcon.

Dr. Jerry D. Cavallerano has no financial or proprietary interest in the materials presented herein.

Dr. Alejandro Espaillat is a consultant for Alcon, Allergan, Ista, Optos, and Elli Lilly.

Dr. Sandra Rocio Montezuma has no financial or proprietary interest in the materials presented herein.

Dr. Timothy J. Murtha has no financial or proprietary interest in the materials presented herein.

Dr. Deval (Reshma) Paranjpe has no financial or proprietary interest in the materials presented herein.

Dr. Roberto Pineda has no financial or proprietary interest in the materials presented herein.

Dr. Jesse Richman has no financial or proprietary interest in the materials presented herein.

Dr. Susannah G. Rowe is a consultant for Allergan and Alcon.

Dr. Cecilia R. Sanchez has no financial or proprietary interest in the materials presented herein.

Dr. Evana Valenzuela Scheker has no financial or proprietary interest in the materials presented herein.

Dr. Sabera T. Shah has no financial or proprietary interest in the materials presented herein.

Dr. Paolo S. Silva has no financial or proprietary interest in the materials presented herein.

Dr. King To has no financial or proprietary interest in the materials presented herein.

Dr. Dorothy Tolls has no financial or proprietary interest in the materials presented herein.

Dr. Glenn C. Yiu has no financial or proprietary interest in the materials presented herein.

Index

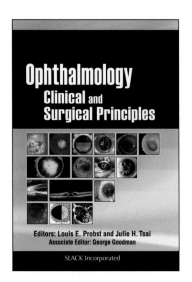
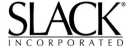